THE
OLDEST GAY
IN THE
VILLAGE

GEORGE MONTAGUE

THE
OLDEST GAY
IN THE
VILLAGE

**A powerful, moving and very
personal account of one man's experience
of being gay over the last nine decades**

JB

JOHN BLAKE

Published by John Blake Publishing Ltd,
3 Bramber Court, 2 Bramber Road,
London W14 9PB, England

www.johnblakepublishing.co.uk

www.facebook.com/Johnblakepub 🖪
twitter.com/johnblakepub 🄴

First published in paperback in 2014

ISBN: 978-1-7821991-6-8

British Library Cataloguing-in-Publication Data:

A catalogue record for this book is available from the British Library.

Design by www.envydesign.co.uk

Printed in Great Britain by CPI Group (UK) Ltd, Croydon, CR0 4YY

1 3 5 7 9 10 8 6 4 2

Papers used by John Blake Publishing are natural, recyclable products
made from wood grown in sustainable forests. The manufacturing processes
conform to the environmental regulations of the country of origin.

Every attempt has been made to contact the relevant copyright-holders,
but some were unobtainable. We would be grateful if the appropriate people
could contact us.

I dedicate this book to the memory of my parents
and my late wife Vera.

With all my love and thanks to my civil partner Somchai,
without whose care and devotion this book would never have
been finished, illustrated or printed.

INTRODUCTION

On Wednesday, 13 July 2013, the Queen affixed her signature to a 64-page document that ended – literally and symbolically – several hundred years of hatred, discrimination and persecution.

The document in Her Majesty's regal hands that day had the catchy title 'Marriage (Same Sex Couples) Act 2013'. Underneath this heading was the explanation that this was 'An Act to make provision for the marriage of same sex couples in England and Wales, about gender change by married persons and civil partners, about consular functions in relation to marriage, for the marriage of armed forces personnel overseas, for permitting marriages according to the usages of belief organisations to be solemnised on the authority of certificates of a superintendent registrar, for the review of civil partnership, for the review of survivor benefits under occupational pension schemes, and for connected purposes.'

Getting this law on to the statute books had been a struggle. It met with implacable opposition from religious groups: more than 400 leading Muslims signed an open letter condemning it on the grounds that they would be robbed of the 'right' to raise their children according to Islamic teaching, while the Bishop of Shrewsbury used his Christmas sermon to equate it with Nazism and Communism.

It also tore apart the Conservative Party, which makes it all the more admirable that Prime Minister David Cameron stuck to his guns, defied his party and pushed the Act through Parliament.

This book is a record of a man's life. A man born in 1923, when homosexuality was not simply despised and misunderstood but was a criminal offence – and one which regularly ruined and imprisoned countless men, young and old.

It is the story of a boy who spent all his childhood in a tiny isolated cottage and left the little village school at the age of 14, barely literate or numerate – but who, thanks to restless energy and a constantly enquiring mind, went on to run his own highly successful business for nearly 50 years.

It is also the story of homosexuality in Britain and of a double-life, of ignorance, intolerance and constant danger. The story of a young man who discovered in his 20s that he was gay, but who married a wonderful woman, fathering three children and – despite living apart from his wife for 22 years – remained extremely close to her until her untimely death.

Britain's legal and institutional hatred of homosexuality would claim many victims – and I was one of them. It led to a cruel and cynical criminal prosecution and the tarnishing of half a lifetime devoted to the Boy Scout movement and to the needs of handicapped children. It would also lead to terrible, and utterly false, suspicions that I was a paedophile.

To call someone a paedophile is to confine them to the lowest circle of hell – and to do so while they are still alive. A convicted paedophile is a 'nonce', and a 'nonce' is the person that every other convicted criminal – burglar, rapist or murderer – can spit on and feel good about it.

Paedophiles are there to be jostled, beaten and shanked (that means raped) in the showers, and the rest of the prison population will whistle and look the other way. It follows that you should not call someone a paedophile unless you are pretty sure of your facts. And certainly not on the basis of crude ignorance and prejudice.

But I am getting ahead of myself.

I don't believe in astrology but it is a lot of fun. My star sign is Gemini, the heavenly twins, and Geminis are said to have a dual nature. I certainly fit that bill and I have come to think of myself as having two sides: 'Gemini A' and 'Gemini B'.

For much of my life I was 'in the closet', hiding my sexuality, living a double life, living a lie, a sort of true-life Jekyll and Hyde. And so, 'Gemini A' is me as most of my friends, Scouting colleagues and business acquaintances knew me. All of them will now have reached late middle age or be even older. Some I hope will read this.

'Gemini B' is the gay me who lived – both covertly and eventually in the open – a good and gay life. All my gay friends will identify with this part. But I also hope members of the general public – particularly those who may have prejudices and homophobic views – will read it and perhaps come to learn something to their (and everyone else's) benefit.

I used to say that where there are prejudices we need to create understanding. But as time has passed I have tended to add we also need acceptance, because we can't expect people to understand what we don't understand ourselves.

For I cannot tell you why I am gay. The one thing that has hurt me and annoyed me more than anything else about being gay is that people will, even to this day, insist on describing it as a 'chosen way of life'.

Can people choose to be left- or right-handed, to be tall or short, to have brown eyes or blue? For years those who were born left-handed were encouraged – and often made – to change. It isn't so long since the colour of a person's hair and eyes was used to determine their 'racial value'. Today we know that for what it was – Nazism and fascism – and we condemn it. So why should anyone think that a homosexual man (or woman, for that matter) should be able to choose their sexuality?

And since they – we – can't, what are we supposed to do about it? Some sections of Christianity like to teach that there is nothing a person who finds that he is gay can do except to be celibate. But why? If he (or she) is true to himself and to others, if this person does no harm – or, at least, no more than a heterosexual person – why should he or she be condemned to a lonely, unhappy life?

I hope that if, as you start this book, you think we have had any 'choice' that by the time you have reached the end of these pages you will have changed your mind; and that you may temper your intolerance with compassion, with sympathy and maybe – just maybe – with understanding and acceptance.

I need to warn you, though. Many of you will find many parts of this account shocking and uncomfortable. There are incidents in it that I regret and others for which I make no apology – however explicitly they may be described. But remember, you are not reading it aloud or discussing it in a group: there is no need for embarrassment, since for the moment it is just this book, you and me.

Nor, of course, do you have to read it all – although I hope you do. For it is a story of its time and for our times.

I am now firmly into my 10th decade on this planet. For too many of them I had to deny who I was – or, at least, to hide a very real part of me from public view. But now, at the age of 91, I am known – celebrated even – for being who I am: within the past few years the Gay Pride March in Brighton (where I have lived for many years) did me the great honour of asking me to lead the parade.

I am the Oldest Gay in the Village. This is the story of my life and, by extension, of countless others; lives lived half in shadow, half in light. And it is also the story of how mine became a love that can finally speak its name.

ONE

On Wednesday, 4 September 1957, a relatively short (just155 pages) government report became an instant bestseller. All 5,000 copies of its first print run sold out within hours of publication. The unlikely sensation had the prosaic, 'A Report on Homosexual Offences and Prostitution', but it would thereafter always be known by the name of the man who headed the committee that drew it up – Sir John Wolfenden.

Wolfenden and 12 other representatives of Britain's great and good had deliberated for three years before arriving at their recommendations. Three years of taking evidence, often in conditions of utmost secrecy, and pondering the nature of homosexuality and what the country should, or should not, do about it.

And when, that morning in September 1957, its

conclusions were finally published they proved revolutionary: 'Homosexual behaviour between consenting adults in private should no longer be a criminal offence.'

It should have been the end: the end of hundreds of years of persecution and prosecution; the end of a modern era in which homosexual men were sent to prison not just for expressing their love but for having that love in the first place. It wasn't, of course. It was, perhaps, a beginning. But for men like me there was a very long and often dark journey to endure before we would be free to think, to feel and to act on our love.

Beginnings. Where do things begin? Where does a story start – especially the story of a man who loves other men? At the beginning, I think: that is where we must start.

I was born on Tuesday, 5 June 1923 at The Mothers' Hospital, Lower Clapton Road, in the poor London borough of Hackney. My mother was 24 and my father seven years older; and since the family home was in Boscombe on the Dorset coast my arrival in the somewhat grimier environs of East London was (and remains) something of a mystery.

My father had trained as a gardener before becoming a policeman. On the outbreak of World War One in 1914 he joined the Grenadier Guards; he was wounded in action before being captured, spending some time as a prisoner of war in Germany.

When the war ended he rejoined the police force and was stationed at Bournemouth, just up the road from Boscombe where my mother was then working as a domestic servant. Strict rules meant that she was not allowed to leave the house except on her night off, so PC Montague would interrupt his duties to court her in true Romeo style from beneath the balcony of the great house where she was in service. Dad was apparently not a good policeman; he was ticked off for being too friendly with the general public. There would come a time – or rather, many times – when I would have cause to wish that other policemen were more like him.

It is one of my great regrets that I never really talked to Mum about her early life: what were her schooldays like? What of her teens – had she had any other boyfriends before Dad? Perhaps I did ask her, but I can't remember her telling me anything. Somehow though, I've always felt that she did not have a happy childhood.

Unusually for those times, her own parents – my maternal grandparents – were separated and Mum had only one brother and no sisters. I never heard about any other relations except for her cousin Auntie Hetty who lived in Reading. We rarely saw her parents; she seldom spoke of them or her childhood and we lost touch completely with her brother.

From the time she married my father, he and all his family and friends became the only relatives she kept in constant touch with. Through Dad she had three sisters-in-law and eventually 12 nephews and nieces, most of whom had offspring. Mum was a real letter-writer and she kept in touch with them all.

I remember very little of my earliest years. Mother later told me that I loved to go up and down in the cliff lift at Boscombe, which cost a halfpenny a time, and that I once sat in Father's police helmet.

But I'm not entirely sure I lived with them: since Mother was working – and since the life of a servant often precluded children in those days – I think I must have spent most of my first three years living with my maternal grandmother in Reading, more than 70 miles away from Boscombe. And in the 1920s, before everyone had a motorcar or even a telephone, 70 miles was an enormous distance. I might as well have been in another country.

Dad left the police force when I was three. The family had just grown in size – my brother Edward was just a few weeks old – when we moved to Hitcham in south Buckinghamshire in the summer of 1926. 'Hitcham House' was the home of the village squire, a wealthy brewer called Colonel Handbury. It was a large traditional country house complete with an estate that included a farm and a typical Victorian walled kitchen garden.

In the centre of this garden was the estate laundry with a tied cottage attached: this was the house in which I was to spend the next 15 years of my life. At the time about 26 servants were employed on the estate, six on the farm and the dairy, about 10 in the house – a butler, two footmen, a cook and kitchen maids, upstairs and downstairs maids – six gardeners, two chauffeurs and an estate carpenter. Mother was taken on as laundress and father as a gardener for four days and was assigned to help mother in the laundry for the remaining two days of the working week (Saturday was a working day in those less enlightened times).

Looking back from the viewpoint that comes with age, I realise just how alien our life must seem to a 21st-century reader. The house was a very old two-up, two-down. There was no bathroom; the toilet consisted of a bucket in a small

4

privy outside, 10 yards from the back door. If it was raining we just had to run for it. And in those days we had long, hard winters with lots of snow and thick ice.

The living room was a little larger than the kitchen, with a single gaslight hanging from the centre of the ceiling. The room had four doors, one in each wall: one led into the kitchen, one into the laundry room, one into a small pantry and the stairs; the other was the front door, which was only opened in the summer. With only a small coal- or log-burning fire, it was very cold and draughty in the winter.

The kitchen was the warmest room in the house and therefore the place where we spent as much time as possible. The centrepiece was a traditional black-leaded cast-iron range: it was heated by a small coal-burning fire and on the removable top plate sat a large black iron kettle. The kitchen fire rarely went out; it was stoked up at night, the damper shut down, then with a tickle in the morning it would flare up to boil the very large heavy kettle for the first of innumerable cups of tea of the day.

Mum did all the cooking in the small oven, with the only means of controlling the temperature being the amount of coal burning in the fire. And yet the food was wonderful: I have lived more than 90 years and apple pie has never been as good as the ones Mum pulled from the basic little range.

The rest of the kitchen was just as primitive. There were no storage cupboards or worktops, just a very well-scrubbed pine table. And, this being long before the days when people had fridges, all the food was kept in the larder under the stairs.

Over the top of the range was the mantelpiece, a long shelf with a short red velvet pelmet and tassels. On this mantelpiece Dad kept his pipes and his tobacco: he always smoked a very strong black shag called Black Beauty; matches and pipe lighters were made by us kids with pieces of tightly rolled newspaper.

Tobacco was the cause of the only disagreement I ever had with my father. When I was grown up I remonstrated with him over smoking. He looked at me and said: 'Son, if you were injured in the front line, the first thing you would ask for would be a cigarette.'

I was a teenager by then and although most of my friends and contemporaries smoked, I never had. It was something about which I felt strongly – and still do: however unconventional (by the standards of the times) my life has been, smoking has never been one of my vices. Which perhaps explains how I have lived so long.

Dad used a small ivory-plated two-bladed knife to dig out the tobacco ash from his pipe: that knife went everywhere him. One day, after noticing how often he used it during a day for cutting and sharpening all sorts of things, we had a conversation and one remark has stayed with me ever since. 'Son, make sure you always have a knife, a piece of string and a sixpence in your pocket.' I still have Dad's little knife: I use it constantly and it, along with the pictures I have of Mum and Dad, is one of my most treasured possessions.

There was little enough entertainment in those cash-strapped and slower days; most winter evenings Dad was to be found in his chair, reading. Of course these hadn't been bought: like most avid readers of our class – and Dad read two or three books a week – they came exclusively from the local free library.

Money, as I say, was tight. There were now six of us living

in the little cottage: my grandmother – Dad's mother – had come to live with us, and from the moment she did I slept with her in the smaller of the two bedrooms, while my baby brother Edward was laid down in a cot in my parents' room. When my sister Betty arrived, Edward and I graduated to a shared bed in a corner of the laundry, screened from the rest of the room by curtains.

We rarely had even a few coppers to spare, and although there were four pubs within a mile of the house we only ever saw the inside of them on special occasions. Dad would nurse a pint of mild and bitter, Mum and my grandmother would have a Guinness or a glass of stout, and we children – treat of treats! – would be given lemonade and a halfpenny currant bun, which was really more like a large biscuit: about three inches square and half an inch thick, very hard and with a only a few currants.

But that's not to say that Dad and Mum went without a drink the rest of the time. All the pubs in those days had a 'Jug and Bottle' where anyone including very young children could go, knock on the 'stable-like half-door', the top half of which only would be opened. On Saturday evenings in the winter, from the age of about eight, I was sent around to The Pheasant, the nearest pub: I would take with me three large plain glass bottles to collect the weekly treat and, if we had been good, a halfpenny bun each for us children.

What we did have, though, was a garden – and it was a reliable, if exacting, source of food for the family. Our cottage had been built on the site of what had once been a very large and very old country house: it had been called Blythewood and I remember it being said that it had been listed in the Domesday book, the 12th-century catalogue of properties of note. Many walls of the old house had been retained as fruit walls and perimeter walls of an enormous kitchen garden.

The whole of this garden was carefully cultivated. Flowers bordered all the many paths behind which grew every conceivable vegetable. On the walls were fruit trees of every kind that would grow outdoors, and in the greenhouses all those that needed heat, such as grapes and figs. On the other side of these walls were two large orchards, one for cherries and the other for apples.

Keeping this neat and tidy was a job that fell to us as children, and I can't say we liked it very much. Still, Mum and Dad were much too poor to give us pocket money so we dug up weeds on the seemingly endless gravel paths to earn some. It was hard work, too: we'd spend entire days down on our knees using an old knife to scrape away the persistent weeds. It made our knees and fingers sore, but I think it taught me a lesson that would be with me all my life: if something needs to be done, then best get on and do it.

I know that Dad spent all the daylight hours of his spare time in the garden, making sure there would be food to put in our hungry tummies. And every day he brought in fresh vegetables: he always grew enough potatoes to last for the whole year and in the summer he dug them fresh every day. And when autumn came and all the remaining potatoes were dug up, we children had to help clean them, then they were put into the corner of the 'coal shed' in a pile covered with straw and sacking. And for all the hard work involved, I can honestly say that I've never tasted better than the first root of very small new potatoes, dug up in the early summer and lightly boiled with a sprig of home-grown mint.

Looking back I know that while we had very little money, unlike many of our contemporaries, we were not really poor: in fact we lived on the fat of the land as far as food was concerned.

You see, although we could never afford to buy meat we never went without it. Dad had a shotgun and the park was teeming with rabbit, hare, partridge and pheasant. Several times a week he would disappear, we would then hear shots and Dad would return with dinner for the next few days.

When I got a little older I used to make wire snares, like a hangman's noose, which I would place in a rabbit run in the long grass, just where they ran under the fence. More often than not, when I went out again just before dark there would be a fat rabbit. If it was not dead I would give it a sharp blow with an open hand, breaking its neck: we never thought this was cruel in those days. It was the only way Dad could feed the family – even the cost of cartridges was a financial problem – and I was glad to do my bit.

And anyway, there were so many rabbits in the park that they were classed as pests: they did a great deal of damage and numbers had to be kept down. Fortunately for us it was not until many years later that the viral disease myxomatosis almost wiped out the total rabbit population: today very little wild rabbit is eaten, but we dined well on it and I learned to skin and paunch rabbits and hares at a very early age.

I was growing, too, into my responsibilities to our family. Once, when I was still a youngish boy, Dad fell ill and Mum bemoaned: 'Oh dear! There is nothing for dinner!' Without telling anyone, I took the gun and having always watched my father I knew just what to do. I approached the warren very slowly and upwind so that the rabbits did not smell me. And I waited for one to appear so I could shoot it.

I remember to this day the recoil kick as the gun went off: it nearly knocked me over, but Dad's good advice – 'Always keep the butt pressed tightly into your shoulder, son' – saved me. I walked tall all the way back home and proudly presented mother with one large rabbit for the pot.

On special occasions we would have a chicken or a cockerel, donated to us from the farm; and on very special occasions such as Christmas we would be given a goose. (We used everything but the goose's honk, as people used to say: even the fat was put into service to grease our boots and protect them from the weather.) But it was many years before I tasted turkey at Christmas: growing up we knew that it wasn't for the likes of us and was reserved for the nobs and snobs in the big house.

The big house, of course, provided not just our living but our home as well. And its demands took an enormous toll, particularly on my mother. My father and mother had more energy and worked harder than any other people I've ever known; from six in the morning till late at night they would be on the go, slaving away in the laundry.

Five and a half days of every week Mum did the washing and ironing for a minimum of 15 people from the big house, where most weekends they would have guests. The washing room was a most unlovely place, with windows on one side only and through which the sun never shone. It had a cold stone floor so that in the winter it was almost freezing unless the coppers (as the water boilers were known) were alight when it would still be nearly as cold but full of smelly steam.

There were two of these coppers: they were large brick-built structures, each with a copper bowl about two feet in diameter, which gave them their nickname. These bowls each held about 10 gallons of water. On the top was a wooden lid and then underneath was a wood-burning fire with an iron door.

Dad used to work in the washing room on Mondays and Tuesdays. Early in the morning before breakfast he would light the fires, fill both coppers by hand with buckets of water then, when they were boiling, in would go the washing, most of which would be white linen. At this point a few handfuls of soda would be added, then this would all be boiled for several hours.

Every now and then Dad would climb a small stepladder and turn the bubbling mass with a three-foot-long stick. I can even now remember the smell of that room.

The next operation was to lift out the two great steaming-hot heavy bundles of washing, which then had to be transferred to several large wooden tubs, where everything would be rinsed again and again in cold water.

With no such thing as spin dryers everything had to be put though the mangle, a large machine with two wooden rollers, one spring-loaded with a handle that turned both rollers, through which the clothes would be squeezed. Those items with buttons on had to be wrung out by hand otherwise the buttons would be broken. All items badly soiled, such as the servants' aprons, shirts collars and cuffs, were scrubbed by hand. I can see Mum and Dad now, bending over the tubs scrubbing away for hours with large brushes using a bar of Sunlight soap.

Tuesdays and Wednesdays were drying days. If it rained for several days, all the washing had to be dried in the drying room. This had two large heavy racks on pulleys hanging from the ceiling; a system of pulleys and cords led down to a windlass on the wall to raise these racks once loaded. In the centre of the room was a cast-iron 'tortoise' – a wood-burning stove which had to be constantly fed with logs.

Unlike the washhouse, the ironing room was a lovely room with a wooden floor about 30-foot square with large windows all along two sides that caught the sun most of the day.

In the centre was a supporting pole that we children used to play around and climb, and all down one side of the room was a 25-foot-long ironing table covered with old blankets and linen. Mother would stand here for hours on end, often late into the evening, doing the enormous heaps of ironing.

Most of the irons were what we called flat irons, about the same size as today's electric ones but in solid cast iron with a steel handle weighing 10 pounds. (I know that because it said so in letters cast into the metal.) These irons were heated on a special square stove with slopping flat sides, with a ridge to hold them steady. The stove was in the corner of the ironing room furthest from the ironing table, and each heated iron would stay hot for only five minutes: that meant constantly going back and forth to reheat them. We worked out that Mum would walk several miles each ironing day.

The reason for the long ironing table was the white linen 30-feet-long tablecloths used at the big house. The gentry there held frequent house parties, dinners and banquets – and the linen had to be both spotless and utterly smooth for each occasion.

When all the washing was finally dry and ironed, it all had to be folded and put into wicker baskets which when full were far too heavy for one person to lift. This process would continue until every item was packed into what became five or six hampers full. This would sometimes take until late on a Friday evening to complete. Then early on Saturday morning a two-wheeled horse-drawn cart would be backed up to the laundry door.

This cart would contain five or six more large hampers full of dirty washing. The baskets with the dirty washing would be unloaded and the clean washing loaded. The dirty washing would straight away be sorted with the very dirty items being put 'in soak', with soda all ready for another week's washing on Monday.

Mum's work didn't stop when she had finished her chores for the big house. In the evenings she would be cooking, preserving fruit, making jams, pickling onions and other produce that Dad brought in from the garden. All the cooking was done on the kitchen range, yet I can honestly say that the standard of her cooking was of the very best: rabbit stew, jugged hare, roast pheasant or partridge, vegetables picked fresh that morning, Brussels sprouts picked with the frost on them – all of it tasted like nectar to our hungry mouths.

The rituals of meal times were religiously observed, as well they might be given how much time and effort had gone into them. Breakfast was always porridge (cornflakes didn't come in until after the war), scrambled eggs on toast and thinly sliced fried potato. Of course there were no such things as electric toasters – we didn't have electricity even if we could have afforded one – so the toast had to be done laboriously with a toasting fork in front of the open fire.

Lunch was a word we never used; the main meal of the

day was dinner at midday. It was many years before I felt comfortable using the word lunch, even when taking my customers out for a midday meal. It felt the same as using the word 'one' when referring to myself: an affectation that belonged to the nobs and snobs not people of our class.

The last meal of the day for us children while still at school was tea: bread and jam and cake, all of which emerged from the doughty range stove. And then it was off to bed.

It's worth remembering in these days of constant hot water and en-suite showers that personal washing was a very different beast in those days. It was achieved – and it *was* an achievement – first thing in the morning and last thing at night using only a large china jug and bowl filled with ice-cold water. We only saw warm water on ironing days.

Mother would call out: 'Don't forget your neck, knees and behind your ears'. If we didn't do it well enough she did it for us – and how it hurt when she did. But lest this sounds like cleanliness wasn't important, I must record that we were sent to wash our hands every time before sitting down at the table, an instruction that was very strictly enforced.

Friday night was bath night. We had an old hip bath into which we put about six inches of water that had been heated on top of the ironing stove in a couple of large heavy cast-iron pots. The ironing room was still warm, the bath was put close to the fire and the clothes racks full of airing clothes were placed around it to form a screen from the draughts. Despite having no bathroom, we children rather enjoyed bath night.

When mother did sit down it would be behind the sewing machine on which she made many of the clothes we wore, including my sister's dresses. If she wasn't working away at our old hand-operated Singer machine, turning the wheel for hour after hour, then she would be knitting, making scarves, socks, gloves and jumpers – most often with wool that she had unpicked from something that was too small, or that she had picked up at a rummage sale.

On the very rare occasions that she bought a new skein of wool, one of us would have to hold it out on our outstretched arms so that she could wind it into a ball. The process made our arms ache. Hardly a night would go by without her darning the heels of a pair of socks, making or mending something or sewing on a few missing buttons.

So why am I telling you all this? What have all these details of a 1920s childhood – a time so remote from today's world that it might as well be on another planet – to do with this story of a man's discovery of his sexuality? Plenty, that's what.

Throughout my life, comedians – amateur and professional – have always told a joke. It runs like this: Two gay men are chatting; one says to the other, 'My mum made me a homosexual'. And the other says, 'If I give her the wool, will she make me one too?' It's a tired old joke and it wasn't all that funny the first time I heard it, but in some way it speaks of an assumption that many – too many – people are far too quick to make: that there must be something in a person's childhood to 'turn' him into a homosexual.

And that's why I've told you all about my years of growing up: I wanted you to see that there was nothing in them to 'make' me gay. No great trauma, nothing wrong with my parents or my family. Maybe now that old, silly theory can be put to bed once and for all, and we can be happy just knowing that sometimes some people are homosexual: they – we, I – just are.

THE OLDEST GAY IN THE VILLAGE

All that said, my childhood years weren't entirely devoid of formative events. In 1934, at the impressionable age of 11, I discovered sex and Scouts – in that order. These two discoveries would dominate my life for decades to come, possibly even until now. And, in one awful twist of unkind fate, they would ultimately and tragically converge.

TWO

I was wearing my Wolf Cub uniform for the last time. It was 1933 and I was about to swap the Cubs' green jersey and peaked cap for the altogether more grown-up uniform of the Scouts: I was 11 years old. I was with a boy who was a little older than me. We had just left the Scout meeting where I had been accepted and inducted into the troop and I was feeling as proud as Punch.

On the way home we were walking though the woods when he jumped up onto a fallen tree, promptly pulled his penis out of his shorts and started masturbating furiously. I didn't know that word then of course, and nor, as far as I can recall, had I ever done what he was doing: it certainly would never have occurred to me to expose myself in front of anyone else, let alone indulge in the sort of remarkably vigorous tugging that my companion was now occupied with.

I was fascinated – the more so when, after a few frantic minutes, I saw a jet of milky liquid come shooting out of his penis. 'How did you do that?' I demanded. I was utterly transfixed – and seeing the evident enjoyment it occasioned, determined that whatever the secret I wasn't going to be left out. It took many months of solitary effort, rubbing myself depressingly and fruitlessly sore, before I experienced my first orgasm. And in that moment I was hooked.

I was still, then, at the same village school where I'd started my education six years earlier. Schooling in those far-off days was rather different to the way it is now: for a start there was only the most rudimentary state school system for children, like me, whose families were poor. Village schools catered for us and gave us as good an education as they could: when adolescence took over from childhood the choices were to pass the examination to go to grammar school or to stay on until we were 14, which was then the leaving age.

I had started school aged five and thoroughly enjoyed my time in the infants: the teacher, a Miss Challen, was young, pretty and I liked her. Then the next year I moved up to Standard One (the class names in those days were as strange as something out of a Victorian school story): the teacher there was a Miss Tanner, who was quite old, very strict, and when she bent down to talk close to you you'd get spit on your face. Perhaps unsurprisingly, I didn't do well at all and when the following year the whole class went up to Standard Two, I had to stay behind: I was, it seemed, a slow learner.

I think I must have had, and to a certain extent still do have, a sort of mild word blindness for although I have never had too much of a problem with reading, I was and still am a very poor speller. I've been told that taking to spelling is something to do with having a photographic memory: I don't have one and I simply can't picture the word in my mind.

But at woodwork, sport and gardening – practical subjects all – I excelled. My biggest problem, though, was shyness, a problem made worse by the fact that I also had a bad stammer. The cause of this was apparently one of the few truly traumatic incidents in my childhood. When I was about three years old I fell into a large circular pond and very nearly drowned. My grandmother saved me, but from that moment on I suffered terribly with stammering.

But my little problem was also the reason I began singing and thereby discovered my truest love affair of all – music. When I was seven years old and walking the mile home from school, I met the wife of my father's then employer; I was very much in awe of her and when I answered her questions I stuttered a great deal even more that usual. Following this encounter she had a word with my mother, telling her to put me in the church choir as singing would cure me of my stuttering: she was right and singing was thereafter to take up a great part of my life.

About this time my family went though a very bad time. My brother Edward caught pneumonia. This developed into double pneumonia. My sister Betty, only a baby at the time, also caught it. The doctor suggested that I be sent away if possible. I was collected by my father's sister, Aunt Gertrude, and whisked off to live with them in London.

It was the first time I had ever been in a car: they had an old Model T Ford and it was, despite all the worries at home, very exciting to rumble along the uncrowded roads from rural Buckinghamshire to Hammersmith.

Aunt Gertrude and Uncle Harry lived in Black Lion Lane. At the end of this road in those days there was a footpath leading down to the Thames and I spent many hours there watching the river traffic. I was particularly fascinated by the pump house, in which sat a huge cast-iron, steam-operated beam engine that pumped London's sluggish water around the city night and day.

Perhaps there is something that connects our childhood experiences with the choices we make in later life. I always remembered the sheer size and power of those huge cast-iron castings – though little did I guess then that I would spend nearly 60 years of my life directly connected to foundries and castings. None, though, were ever as impressive to me as that large old beam engine.

My brother was ill for a long time: he nearly died – twice – but my family refused to give up hope. Mother and grandmother between them fought his illness until he turned the corner and got well. Then I was allowed to go home.

But within a month of being back, another of my aunts begged my Mum to let me go and stay with her. Auntie Hetty and Uncle Tom had never been able to have children of their own and, after a little discussion, I was sent down to Reading to stay with them.

It was at Reading that I first developed my love of classical music. The house boasted a wind-up gramophone and 12-inch 78rpm records of Strauss, Beethoven, Chopin, Bach and the composer who would come to be my favourite: George Frideric Handel. I have lived with, and loved, this music now for more than 80 of my 90 years and, whenever I hear it, I think of Auntie Hetty and Uncle Tom and my time with them in Reading where I first heard and was captivated by it. And

I remember, too, that when, after four months, it was time for me to go home Auntie Hetty cried.

So, aged eight, I returned to the little tied cottage and the closeness of my family. We lived very near to the village church and, in the hope that it would help my stammer, I joined the church choir. I was, in truth, too young and also so behind with my schooling that I could hardly read. But they were short of boys and so I was swiftly issued with a cassock – even the shortest was much too long. But I was thrilled, and to make it even better I discovered that I was to be paid for singing.

The vicar was a wise and kindly man; a great character who would have a great influence on my early years. It was he who first told my family that Montague was a very noble name. Little did I know that nearly 20 years later I would discover I shared more than ancestry with a peer of the realm.

In spite of what I am about to recount these were, I think, more innocent times: certainly the way boys and girls interacted – or didn't – was very different than the way children grow up today. In the 1930s boys had to wear shorts, no matter what the weather, until the day they left the village school at the age of 14. And until we left school we had absolutely nothing to do with girls.

It wasn't that girls didn't inhabit the same space as us – there were 15 boys and 15 girls in our little village school – but it was an unwritten and inviolable rule that all the boys sat together in class. And that closeness led, inevitably, to sexual experimentation.

There was a great deal of group masturbation amongst us boys. We thought nothing of it, but at the same time we made sure no girl (let alone an adult) saw us. It would even happen in the school classroom and occasionally during class time. It would happen in church when, as choirboys during the sermons and in full view of the congregation with our surplices stretched tight over our knees we learned to wank ourselves off (and sometimes each other) without a single ripple being visible. Looking back I realise that the risk of discovery must have been part of the thrill we experienced.

There was no sex education for children at all in those days: no books or pamphlets of any kind mentioning the subject (if there had been, I'm sure someone would have discovered them and they would have been eagerly sought after and passed around).

No adult, schoolteacher, Scout leader, parent or priest ever mentioned the subject of sex, except to issue dire warnings about the perils of self abuse: 'You will grow hairs in the middle of your hand' or 'You will go blind' was the limit of our adult-instilled understanding of sex. So powerful were these admonitions that we did worry about the consequences of our pleasure, often closely examining the palms of our hands for telltale signs of impending doom. But even this failed to put a kink in our discovery of pleasure.

I don't believe that our eager adoption of mutual masturbation meant we were gay – not that the word had been claimed by homosexuals back then. As far as we were concerned, the word gay meant colourful, happy and outgoing. Nor had we ever heard of the labels 'homosexual' or 'queer', and if even if we had I doubt we would have known what they meant.

For those, like me, who were in the Scouts there was the additional burden of knowing that we were wilfully flouting the strictures laid down in the organisation's bible. Baden-

Powell laid down the rules in his book *Scouting For Boys*: to me this was a far more important text than the Bible itself, and Baden-Powell was absolutely clear that masturbation (let alone mutual wank sessions) was absolutely forbidden. According to B-P, it was 'unclean and unmanly' and something that only a cigarette-smoking weakling would give in to. And the advice on how to resist this terrible temptation? Go and have a cold shower.

Well, I wasn't a cigarette smoker and was quite clear in my own mind that I wasn't a weakling, but I simply couldn't forego the satisfaction to be achieved at my own hands. I'm sure there were some Scouts, perhaps those who had a low sex drive, who could refrain and would be satisfied with nocturnal emissions. I too had these wet dreams, but for me and many of my contemporaries you might as well have told us to stop going for a pee as to cease masturbating.

Still, that's as far as any of this went. Nothing more serious ever happened than what we called 'Bashing the Bishop'. And we were utterly ignorant of the mechanics of sex: one day when walking home from school, I heard some older boys shouting: 'Whip it in, whip it out and wipe it!' I recall very clearly thinking about this in some puzzlement: surely they must have meant: 'Whip it out, wipe it then whip it in'? Even after thorough consultation with my friends and fellow onanists, this remained a mystery: it would be a long time before we worked out what it meant.

Practically all the boys who left the village school at the same time as myself were either in the Scouts, the choir, or both, so we continued to see a great deal of each other. I would get together with quite a number of these for mutual sexual relief, though usually only two of us at a time. Very little was said about what we were doing and nothing at all was ever disclosed to anyone else.

We talked a lot about girls and now and again one would boast that he had, 'done it'. I felt very envious but I never know whether to believe this: having actual sex with an actual girl was something so remote from our little world that I couldn't quite believe it happened. I must have been in my early to mid-teens when I had my first taste of pornography.

In these modern, connected days, when explicit images and films are available via the privacy of a computer and with the simple click of a mouse, it is difficult to grasp just how protected we were from any sort of sexualised images. Nonetheless, a magazine came into my teenage possession and it marked the start of a realisation that my enjoyment of sexual activity with other men might not be a simple issue of convenience and availability. The magazine was called *Health and Efficiency*. It was, ostensibly at least, about naturism and showed full frontal pictures of nudists (albeit with their public regions frequently airbrushed to invisibility). I would keep this treasure carefully hidden, only getting it out at bedtime for perusal during my regular 'going to sleep masturbation'.

From the outset I realised – and was initially puzzled – that I got more turned on by looking at the photographs of a man's penis than at the vaginas of the ladies. What could this mean? Simultaneously something was changing within my group of friends: most of them no longer wanted to 'play around together' (as we chastely described our mutual masturbation sessions). I still wanted to but they, without actually saying anything, tactfully avoided my advances.

They were, in short, beginning to discover girls; and, it must be said, so was I.

On one occasion a number boys and girls were larking around together. It was all fairly harmless until it was suggested that we play 'kiss chase'. This involved the girls chasing the boy of their choice and kissing him (how innocent and childlike this seems today). A girl named Joy caught me and I ended up sitting on her knee being kissed. It was the first time I had been kissed on the lips by anyone and I rather enjoyed it. I duly got an erection.

Did I realise then what this presaged? I doubt it, somehow: I don't think the teenage George Montague could have foreseen any of the alarums and excitements that would befall me in later years. And anyway, life had suddenly become hectic: I was simply much too busy for introspection (even if I could have spelled it).

I finished my schooling soon after my 14th birthday. I could never have passed the grammar school exam and must have come very near to, if not bottom of, the class. And so I left the little village school barely literate or numerate.

These were the 1930s – 'the Hungry Thirties' – where economic depression and unemployment stalked the length and breadth of the land (and indeed much of the world). In those pre-welfare state times there was no unemployment pay or social security and a record number of adult men were unemployed, on short time, or had had their wages cut: millions of families throughout Britain came close to starvation – and many of those did actually go without food for lengthy periods.

But if there was no work for adult men, there were jobs to be found by 14-year-old boys: we, after all, cost a great deal less to employ than a skilled man who had children to feed. And so, for me and most of my friends leaving school was less a choice than a necessity: life – adult life – demanded that we get a job and help out with the family finances.

In truth, most of us were pleased to walk away from education – not least because we would now be able to wear long trousers. I had bought my own pair with my own money – earned by delivering newspapers – before I left school. But until the day I walked out of the school gate for the last time I had only been allowed to wear them on Sundays.

So what did life in the grown-up world hold for young George Montague? Well, as luck would have it, it held a holiday – of a sort. From the beginning of August to halfway though September each year the whole of the family up at the big house – complete with maids, servants, grooms and chauffeurs – migrated to a shooting lodge in Scotland for the annual grouse and stag shoot.

The lady of the house had seemingly taken an interest in me and offered me (through my parents) a job as a 'pony boy' on the shoot. And I jumped at the chance.

On the day we left we all went very early to Taplow railway station. There, a special carriage was waiting, half of which was First Class and the other half Third Class. We were assigned our seats according to our station in life.

It took all day to get to the lodge, deep in the Trossachs. But however tired the journey had made me I was thrilled at the sight of the lochs and the mountains – Ben Lomond, Ben Ledi and Ben Venue. As the weeks progressed I would climb them all and would fish the lochs for pike.

The shooting weeks took on their own particular routine. Each day we rose very early and headed up into the mountains where the gentry would first stalk and then shoot the deer. My job was to lead a pony, following the hunt at a good distance and then, when a kill had been made and the stag had been loaded on to my mount, I would lead it down and follow them home. There were three ponies altogether: rarely were there fewer than two stags shot, and sometimes we brought home three.

As the weeks progressed I learnt a great deal about preparing game, plucking and paunching the birds, skinning the deer and preparing the fish caught in the lochs. I had been assigned a chaperone, presumably because I was just 14, for the adventure: it turned out to be Mrs Wilder, the cook.

And there was a lot to learn. After the 12th of August our quarry would be grouse, blackcock and snipe. To this day I remember feeling sad when the skins and the heads of the deer, minus the antlers – cut off as trophies – were dumped into a large pit. And I was mightily surprised when the grouse were hung until they were lousy with maggots before being plucked and cooked.

Looking back I can see that I was very lucky to have been able to have such a 'holiday', which even though I worked – and worked hard – is how I viewed it. And there was another reason the trip stuck in my memory: I received my first taste of oral sex.

There were three Scottish lads helping out with our party. They lived in cottages at the hunting lodge, sons of the men who were the beaters – the men who drove the birds towards the guns. These boys were about the same age as me, so I spent a great deal of my time with them: we quickly became friends and when I was not working we would play about together.

Being a strange-speaking Sassenach (as they cheerfully termed the English) I was bound to get a ragging: this took the form of a mass rough and tumble in a hayloft. They held me down on the floor and at one point one of them said, 'Let's get 'is wee winkle oot.' They duly freed my small penis from my trousers and then – to my surprise and, at the time, disgust – one of them sucked it.

It would be very many years before I experienced oral sex again. Years in which I would become involved, emotionally and sexually, with a woman; and years in which the circumstances for men who were attracted to other men would become increasingly difficult and downright hostile. But first there would be the little matter of a world war to contend with.

On my return from Scotland I knew that I had to get a job. I was determined not to go into domestic service like my parents. I was not what you might call politically aware and, of course, it would be many years before I was old enough to vote, but if I could have, I would unquestionably have voted Labour. I had grown up living in and surrounded by the aristocracy, and I hated it.

I hated the servility that my parents had to show to their employers; I hated the knowledge that we children had to hide indoors if ever the 'nobs' (as we called them) came around. If and when they did, my father and mother were always addressed, patronisingly to my mind, by their surname, and Dad touched his hat when addressed. I hated, too, the rules of my parents' employment: if either Dad or Mum lost their job then we would have had to leave the tied cottage within one week. And I saw the fruits of privilege every day: Eton College, the snobbiest of all snobs' schools, was nearby: I hated the boys there and their parents to boot.

Instead, I headed down to the local Youth Employment office, where I was asked what I wanted to do. I told them I was good at woodwork and suggested that being a woodworker might suit me. It wasn't long before I was sent to see a prospective employer. Mr Brett ran his business from a private house using his large garage. On the day I called, his wife showed me to an outhouse where Mr Brett was cutting a piece of wood on a circular saw. Without looking up he said: 'What do you want?' I told him I wanted a job. To which he replied: 'What makes you think you could be a patternmaker?'

I probably just looked at him with my mouth open: I had never heard of patternmaking and had no idea what it involved (to the best of my adolescent knowledge, patterns were what mother used to make up my sister's dresses). Mr Brett took me into the workshop, then his phone rang and he disappeared to answer it. But he also told me I could start on a month's trial.

I went home in something of a daze and announced the good news to my mum. And it turned out to be very good news indeed, and to be one of the very many lucky days of my life. Woodworking – by which I mean cabinet making and joinery – would shortly become largely mechanised, but patternmaking was a highly skilled and well-paid job requiring a great deal of handcraft. A good patternmaker was never out of a job. That was a fact then and it's still true to this day. My accidental apprenticeship with Mr Brett would, in time, lead me to my own successful business.

The terms upon which I was engaged involved five years as an apprentice, to be followed by two years as 'an improver'. During the following weeks I discovered that the craft I had fallen into was very highly skilled, akin to engineering in wood: but it also included being a woodwork specialist and model maker.

The wages for a fully qualified 'journeyman' (as a skilled craftsman was known) patternmaker were then two shillings and sixpence and hour – the equivalent to 13 pence in modern currency. Most other skilled workers only received two shillings, with unskilled workers getting just one shilling an hour. But I quickly discovered two unpleasant facts about my new employer.

The first was that he was more interested in getting me to do all sorts of odd jobs than in teaching me my trade: I had to clean his car, work in his garden and clean out the large cage of budgerigars he kept in his house. The second was that he was a 'chain' smoker, the first I had ever known. He used just one match a day, constantly lighting each new cigarette from the stub-end of the previous one. At least twice a day, and sometimes three times, he would send me to the shop at the end of the road with one shilling (five pence) to feed into a slot machine; this would then disgorge a packet of 20 Players cigarettes, with a halfpenny piece change inside the packaging.

To my disgust, Mr Brett coughed constantly and would sometimes spit great blobs of revoltingly coloured phlegm onto a piece of sandpaper. Nor did food slow down his appetite for tobacco: while he was eating he alternated between one mouthful of food and one drag on his cigarette.

Still, with the benefit of hindsight – and despite the way he treated me – I have one thing to thank him for. At a time when nobody knew the dangers, almost every adult male (and very many adolescent boys) smoked. I never did: Mr Brett's disgusting ritual of inhaling and expectorating was enough to put me off for life.

I stayed at Brett's for about a year until one day, while cycling to work, I started chatting to another lad about the same age as me. He was also an apprentice patternmaker and he told me that he was working for the only other 'Master Pattern Maker' in the area. What was more, his apprenticeship including going to night school three evenings a week. I decide then and there to leave Mr Brett's smoky employ. A few weeks later I was taken on at The Machine Pattern Company Ltd and I knew I had made the right decision for my future.

There were about 10 good craftsmen, a great deal of machinery and one other apprentice younger than I was, so I did not have to do any 'shop jobs' such as sweeping up and making the tea. I started attending night school three nights a week to study English, Maths and Technical Drawing. I studied hard, did extra work at home and in the next three years learned more than in all the years I had spent at the village school.

But there were clouds on the horizon. War was coming and a big, all-consuming war at that. It started in the year that I turned 16. I was enjoying my job very much but most lads of my age were already set on joining the forces, flying airplanes, going overseas to fight for King and country. The minimum age for enlisting was 17 and a half. When I reached that milestone I decided to volunteer since I realised I would be called up at 18 anyway.

I was interviewed at the Reading recruiting office and accepted. The following morning I gave in my notice to my employers, who I thought would be proud of me for wanting to 'do my bit'. Instead my boss was furious, and brusquely informed me that I was in a 'reserved occupation'. Patternmakers were, of course, in great demand for a war that would be fought with mechanised armour.

My boss contacted the RAF and I duly received a letter confirming what he had said: my enlistment was refused because I was working as an apprentice patternmaker. If, however, I quit my job, the RAF promised they would re-accept me after a waiting period of three months.

I was furious. I wanted to serve my country in its time of need, not skulk about in a reserved occupation – no matter how important it might be to the war effort. I handed in my notice and took a job at the Hawker Aircraft Company three miles away: here they were building and repairing crashed Hurricane fighter planes shot down in the Battle of Britain.

Ever since then Hurricanes have always been my favourite aircraft. People think that the Spitfire won the Battle of Britain, but there were four Hurricanes to every Spitfire. I worked in the repair department where crashed and damaged planes were repaired or rebuilt, and I was proud to do so.

It was a six-mile bicycle ride from home to the factory so, when they asked for volunteers for fire watching – bombing of aircraft factories was high on the Luftwaffe's agenda – I jumped at the chance. I stayed at the works three nights a week and also some weekends. There were about six of us all about the same age who took it in turns to patrol the factory and surrounding airfield in pairs.

There was an added benefit in that we had free use of an

old Armstrong Siddeley car that was kept on the airfield. Several of us taught ourselves to ride and drive, crashing up and down its primitive pre-synchronisation gearbox. But the war was growing ever more murderous and I realised it was time to shoulder a bit more of the burden. In September 1941, at the age of 18, I enlisted in the Royal Air Force Volunteer Reserve: it was the start of a journey which would take me halfway round the world – and which would rudely re-awaken the sleeping giant of my sexuality.

THREE

'Montaeg! What are you doing there?'

We were lined up on the tarmac of an RAF base at Warrington in Lancashire. The line had been formed on the somewhat arbitrary principal of foot size: although I was not particularly tall – just five feet nine in my stockinged feet – I have always had large feet, and duly positioned myself between young men much taller than me. It must have looked absurd – at least that's what the sergeant who was now yelling at me thought – while completely mispronouncing my name.

'I've got big feet sarge – size ten and a half. Oh, and my name is Mon-ta-gue.' I was learning the hard way that the military doesn't cope well with the unexpected or unusual: it's a wonder he didn't tell me I must do some fat-i-gue. There were no half sizes. I was issued with size 11 and told to get on with it.

A few weeks earlier I had received a form from the recruiting office at Reading, informing me that I had been accepted as a trainee wireless operator air gunner in the RAF volunteer reserve. During the short time I spent at Warrington I was issued with the full set of flying equipment: flying suit, fur-lined boots, fur-lined gloves with silk inner gloves, helmet and goggles. I was also given a small white flash which fitted into my forage cap, indicating that I was trainee aircrew. I was 18 and there were three things uppermost in my mind: to be posted overseas, to fly in an airplane and to lose my virginity – with a girl, of course.

The war and joining up had done nothing to dampen my rampant interest in sex: I still masturbated two, three, sometimes four times a day. Sometimes I would be overcome with shame and try not to: I would avoid going to the toilet for as long as I could, as I would, once installed in the latrines, be overcome with the need to do it again. But these attempts at abstinence never lasted long – and the objects of my fantasies when taking myself in hand were always female.

I had been in the RAF several months when I first heard the expression 'brown hatters'. I had no idea what it meant, but on listening further to the conversations of my fellow recruits I gathered it meant men who had sex with men. There was a distinct hostility among the ranks to this, and those who were afflicted (for this was how it was viewed) by such desires were dismissed with the vituperative label 'homos'; it was the first time I had ever heard that expression, too.

One of the other recruits announced: 'I've got one, I think, in my hut'; another said: 'I think I've got two in mine – if I ever catch them together I'll cut their bollocks off.' And I think I was as guilty of this unthinking prejudice as everyone else. After a little discreet questioning I discovered exactly what these hated homos got up to – and I was genuinely just as disgusted and shocked as the others were. Nothing was further from my mind at that time than that I might be homosexual myself.

We were eventually posted to Blackpool to do our square bashing, as foot drill was universally known. We were all billeted in one of the small three- or four-storied guesthouses. Our landladies were very strict and very stingy with the food – though since rationing was in full force I imagine they had to be. They gave us very thin slices of ready-buttered bread: in reality this meant that they had spread the butter over its surface – and then scraped it all off again. We had to spend some of our very small weekly pay packet on fish and chips just to keep our strength up.

Drill was done in the street in squads of about 24, each under the instruction of a master instructor. Two of these were very well known in the entertainment world and became even more renowned after the war. Max Wall and Max Miller were famous comedians doing their bit for Britain: I was in Max Wall's squad.

Every weekday after about an hour's drill we were marched into the town to the huge bus and tram sheds. These were set out with tables and chairs to seat 12; each was equipped with headphones and a Morse code tapping key. The instructor would tap out sets of four digits and numbers at an ever-increasing speed that we then had to decode and write down.

I thought I had a head start on most of the others for I had learned the Morse code in the Scouts. The qualifying speed was 18 words a minute, which I could just about managed to achieve. But before the exam they increased the rate to 24 words a minute. I think they had too many applicants for aircrew.

Despite practising more than most of the other lads, my brain simply wouldn't concentrate sufficiently and I was unable to cope. To my immense shame I was taken off the course: I had to leave all the friends I had made, hand back all my flying kit, take out the special white aircrew trainee flash from my cap and then think about what I was going to do instead.

At the time it was a bitter disappointment to me, but looking back I realise that I was lucky: had I been successful I might not have survived the war because a large percentage of air gunners and wireless operators were killed.

I had always been interested in sport. So I applied, and was accepted, for training as a Physical Training and Drill Instructor. I was posted to Arbroath on the east side of Scotland, and for the first few days we polished up on our parade drill. Then we were instructed how to command and control a squad of 20 men in complicated drill manoeuvres.

The base had a huge parade ground and we had to march the men several hundred yards away while giving them audible instructions to move to the left, to the right, double march, slow march, about turn and innumerable other drill commands.

Just like children at school the men were not very kind to each other; we all played up and made it as difficult as we could for anyone who wasn't confident or who did not shout loud enough, even if we could hear him.

The most important asset of a good drill instructor is his voice: the archetypal sergeant major yelling at his squad. If one is nervous then this shows, the voice becomes a squeak with no volume. I was a quiet, shy country boy in those days and my squad was a complete shambles. I knew exactly what I should be doing and how to do it, but I was a bundle of nerves. I was the worst instructor on the parade ground and the lads were forever laughing at me – until the day that changed my life. Humiliated, with eyes full of tears, I suddenly got mad. Instead of a feeble peep, my orders emerged from my mouth with a very loud and clear bass voice. That was the day I found my self-confidence.

The first hurdle was over; those of us who had passed the course were posted to South Wales for a period of three months on a physical training course. This involved eight hours a day of intense activity and gymnastics in a very large gym. We learned how to lay out, control, judge and referee all field, track events and sports. We had to run a couple of five-mile and one 15-mile cross-county races most weeks. In the evenings we were given lectures on anatomy and physiology, then in what was left of the day we had to write up notes on all of it.

When it comes to building a healthy, fit but not over-developed body I think the most crucial years are 18 to 23. I exercised thoroughly and daily, keeping myself in tip-top condition. I'm sure the foundations of the health, fitness and energy which have served me in good stead ever since (no matter what I occasionally threw at it) were laid then – and I consider myself extremely lucky.

One of the proudest days of my life up until then was the day I was told I had passed. I was immediately promoted to full corporal and given a badge indicating that I was a Physical Training & Drill Instructor. I was then given leave and told that I would be reporting back to Liverpool. I knew what this meant – an overseas posting.

On 14 August 1943 I returned to Liverpool and, together with 4,000 other men, embarked the SS *Orduna*, a converted meat refrigeration ship pressed into war service. We were not told where we were going, but those like me who had been in the Scouts knew we were heading west. We thought this was strange, wondering if, for some obscure military reason, we were being sent to America, but after two days the *Orduna* turned a large and lazy half-circle and pointed her bow east.

We were told later that the purpose of this manoeuvre was to avoid submarines in the Bay of Biscay. We were the first convoy to sail through the Mediterranean following the end of the fighting in North Africa and fighting was still going on in Italy. Sure enough, we were dive-bombed and one of the ships in the convoy was hit: however, it didn't sink and I once again wondered about my apparently continuing streak of good luck.

We slipped into the Suez Canal and anchored up at Port Said: almost instantly we were surrounded by small boats full of young men trying to sell us souvenirs. Not many of us bought anything, but just over three years later when we were on our return trip I would have cause to remember the eagerness of these youths – and their willingness to sell us almost anything.

We reached our initial destination – Durban at the foot of South Africa – on 14 September: we had been at sea for 31 days. For 10 days we were put into huts, if you could call them that: four walls made of sacking with large holes but no windows; two large doorways but no doors. When it came to bedtime I noticed that the lads had put their shoes one under each of two of the bed legs, with their kit bags locked and trapped by the handle under another leg. When I enquired as to why, I was told that during the night local youths – completely naked and covered in grease – would run through and pick up any thing not fixed down. Throughout the 10 days, we lay in wait for our visitors. Once, we even managed to grab one of them, but because of the grease smeared over his body we couldn't hold on to him.

And then we were off again, on to our final destination – an RAF base at what was then called Salisbury in the neighbouring country of Rhodesia – now renamed Harare and Zimbabwe respectively. The camp consisted of a large airfield, with about 75 aircraft, 150 trainee pilots and a total of 1,500 men on camp. I was the third and most junior member of the sports team.

In those days almost everyone smoked – and whereas in England a packet of 20 Players was one shilling (5p) here they were nine old pennies (4p) for a packet of 50 – the least you could buy. The first thing the head of the team asked me was whether I smoked. I don't think he believed me when I said no, because he warned me that if he ever I found me with a cigarette I would be instantly kicked off the team.

It was an important and vital encouragement: the atmosphere in camp was resolutely macho and it was widely believed that if you didn't smoke, you would not drink, nor have sex with girls – in other words you were one of the dreaded band of homosexuals. With all the ribbing and teasing I received from my squad mates I might eventually have succumbed. Thanks to the warning ringing in my ears I resisted the pressure of my peers.

The nearest town was one hour's drive away on what we called 'the liberty wagon', a rattling old canvas-backed army lorry with bench seats that weren't fixed down and which would rudely eject their passengers if the driver took corners too fast. The road itself was equally basic: two concrete strips about a foot wide. This would have been fine for an average car but at the back of our liberty wagon only one of the double wheels was on the concrete. This might not have been so hazardous if the rains had not washed away the surrounding earth: often there was a perilous six-inch drop either side of the strip. Trips into town were, as a result, not for the faint-hearted.

On one of my trips into town, I saw a notice offering driving lessons and the issue of a Rhodesian driving licence. I went in and found that the one person there was both the instructor and also the examiner. I told him that I could drive, but didn't have a British licence. He wasn't worried and, after adding on an extra fee for the use of his ancient Morris, I was sent out to begin my instruction. I expected him to close up his office and come with me, but instead he just stood in the doorway and told me to keep driving around the block until he signalled me to come in.

After less than an hour I was issued with my Rhodesian driving licence: I would never take a British driving test because on my return to the UK all I had to do was show the hastily-issued Rhodesian document and I was presented with a full and permanent British version.

Hiring a car in Salisbury was very cheap and I began to

exploit my new found freedom as often as possible, which is how I finally lost my virginity – and my innocence.

I had been in Rhodesia for a few months and had come to realise that, with 60,000 RAF personnel – all men, there being no WAAFs (Women's Auxiliary Air Force) – in a country with a population with the same number of white people, I was unlikely to find myself walking out with a white girl.

And in truth this didn't bother me. Although Rhodesia was a country founded on racism and the culture of Britain was, at best, casually dismissive of coloured people, I had never felt that prejudice. It was, perhaps, another manifestation of my intolerance of the old English superiority complex that I had found so disgusting in the attitudes of the gentry at the big house at home.

And so when, one weekend, I met a girl whose father had been a Scotsman, but her mother had been black, it seemed to me the most natural thing in the world to go to bed with her. Her name was Ann, and she was about the same age as me. But although I lost my virginity that evening, it was evident that hers had departed long before. She was very experienced, certainly compared to someone whose only experience of sex was largely solitary masturbation. The evening was an extraordinarily powerful experience and while I don't think I fell in love with Ann, I did become very fond of her indeed.

Ann was very poor, living in just one small room in a small house. Although she had a job, I gave her some money each time I saw her: was this a sort of prostitution – a commercial as well as quasi-romantic relationship? I'm not sure. I don't believe she went with any other men during the year that I was with her. The Air Force largely turned a blind eye to what I and my fellow servicemen got up to. Only once, when we were training for a weightlifting competition, did I receive any firm instructions about sexual activity – and even that was more in the way of sporting advice.

That morning the senior officer called us together: 'Now I know some of you have girlfriends in the town,' he pronounced. 'But don't get into bed with them before the show.'

Now I rarely had sex with Ann fewer than three times a night – and that was if I only spent the evening with her. If I spent the entire night you could double that tally. I thought about my superior's advice, and decided to ignore it. I made love to Ann twice that same afternoon – and went on to achieve a personal best at the weightlifting competition in the evening. So much for abstinence.

After a year together I was posted to a base a long way away from Salisbury. It meant that I would no longer be able to see Ann, and an end to our sexual adventuring. The new base was up country and it wasn't until 12 months later that I managed to get a flight with one of the instructor pilots back to Salisbury. We only had about a couple of hours on the ground – just time enough for me to go to see Ann.

When I got there she was out, but her room was open. I went in and waited, hoping she would return before I would have to set off back to the airfield. While waiting I noticed there was evidence of a baby in the room. Just before I thought I would have to leave she returned, carrying a baby on her hip. The words were out of my mouth before I could even say hello: 'Whose baby?' She was coy, replying only, 'He's mine.'

I looked at the little boy. He was whiter than her, but with enough of her colouring to convince me. 'He's nine months old,' she said. And then she guessed my next question and answered it before I could ask. 'Yes, it's yours.'

My immediate feeling was one of guilt. But during the next few minutes she convinced me that she was quite happy. She now had a local boyfriend. He was in the army and was supporting her, and he accepted the baby as his own. There was nothing I could do, she told me – and then proceeded to inform me that both she and her new lover were happy that her son was whiter than they were. I found that almost impossible to understand, but talking to colleagues later I came to realise that this was all too typical – a symptom of the racism that held Rhodesia in its unforgiving grip.

Naturally I have thought about Ann and my son many times in the decades that have passed. I am filled with sadness that I can't remember if she told me his name, and I have always regretted that I have no photograph of them.

One of the oddities of life on an RAF base somewhere so remote from the carnage engulfing the rest of the world was that we didn't really consider the progress of the war and what was going on in Europe or Asia. And even if we had been desperate to do so it would have been almost impossible: there were no radios and, of course, no television. We got to know the major happenings through the informal servicemen's grapevine: and for the rest of our time we were, I'm faintly ashamed to say, too busy enjoying ourselves in the sun, playing sport at every opportunity during the day and dutifully drinking cheap beer in the evenings.

But that wasn't to say that the future wasn't on our minds. During my last months in the RAF my thoughts were increasingly focused on getting home, getting a job, finding a girlfriend and getting married. I bought several presents that I promised myself I would give to my future wife. And then, at last, in May 1945 it was VE day: the war in Europe was over – and we would be going home.

Within a month, two-thirds of all the men on camp were sent back to Blighty. Everything was organised according to your enlistment number: the earlier you had joined up, the lower your number. Those with later numbers – and that included me – watched with envy as the 'on the boat' parties left the camp. But finally, almost a year later, my day came: I was on the boat and on the way home. I left camp on Tuesday, 20 August 1946 – almost three years exactly from the day I had arrived in Rhodesia. But when we arrived once again in Durban and looked for the ship that would carry us back to Britain, we were very disappointed to be told we would be stuck there for three more weeks. In fact, it turned out to be a month – four agonising weeks that felt like the longest month of my life. There was nothing to do, no sporting facilities whatsoever. Nothing to keep me occupied but thoughts of home and family and, so I hoped, the chance at last to meet a girl with whom I could settle down.

We finally embarked the SS *Maloja* on 19 September 1946, bound for Southampton via numerous stopping-off ports along the route. Our first stop was Mombasa, on the southernmost shores of Kenya, and it was here that the jerky voyage of my sexuality encountered a new, and prophetic, interruption.

We were given several hours' shore leave to spend touring the town. As I wandered through the narrow streets a very handsome Kenyan young man, about 19 or 20 years old, came up to me and whispered: 'Would you like to have my sister, boss? My sister very pretty.'

I had not had sex for some time and so I agreed eagerly. I followed him; we made our commercial transaction and I 'had' his so-called 'sister'. When I came out of the little house where we had coupled I found the young man waiting for me. I thought he was about to demand more money but instead he asked if I had enjoyed his 'sister'. I said – honestly, if not exactly gallantly – that it had been okay.

It seemed this young man wanted to talk to me, and so we sat down on a seat overlooking the docks and began chatting. His English was broken but quite extensive. He asked me all about England and then asked whether I had a girlfriend back home. I told him that I hadn't – though I hoped to.

He moved closer to me; his hand was on my knee and he was looking straight into my eyes and I somehow knew he wanted sex with me. I had just had sex with his 'sister', but I had an erection and I realised I also wanted him. I was totally confused. In a daze I said I had to get back to the boat, and made a bolt for it. We sailed shortly after, with my mind still in turmoil. But of one thing I was certain: had we not pulled out of Mombasa I would have gone back to look for the enticing and unnerving young man. For days I worried over the encounter. I'm sure somehow he must have known I also wanted him. But how? How did he know? And what on earth was the matter with me anyway – wanting to have sex with another man?

In the end something happened that helped to take my mind off the young man and my sexual dilemma: I had a terrible itching in my pubic hairs. I told a close friend who inspected my groin and announced: 'You've got crabs – pubic hair lice.'

I was horrified: my tawdry encounter with the young man's 'sister' had resulted not just in turning my emotions inside out but in the acquisition of some kind of sexual passengers. To make it worse, these were the days before the availability of an ointment to encourage these unwanted visitors to depart. My friend grinned as he saw my embarrassment: 'Don't worry. All you have to do is shave all the hairs off.'

I know that today the shaving, sculpting and waxing of pubic hair is a fashion statement and discussed openly. But in 1946 the only reason to take a razor to your private parts was because you'd got lice. It felt shaming – and it had a lingering effect since once the hairs started to grow again it felt like walking with a man's stubble-haired chin clamped between your legs. I should, perhaps, have learned a lesson. But I didn't – as we shall see.

I woke up on Monday, 7 October and peered out of the porthole. We were passing the Isle of White – home! – and what struck me most was how green the grass was. As we docked in one of the large quays at Southampton, the dockside was deserted except for a small group of people and a small child. As we got closer I was amazed to recognise my sister Betty, the small child I realised must be my new little sister Margaret whom I had never seen, and my mother.

I rushed to the gangway, but was told by the military police that I could not go ashore. All those lining the side of the ship shouted, 'Let him off!' and an officer grudgingly agreed, 'Go on then, 10 minutes only.' Mum, as usual was at the back of the group, so the first one I embraced was Betty, who was holding my little sister Margaret's hand. After 10 minutes I got back on board – to discover that my shipmates all thought my sisters were my wife and small daughter.

It was four days later before I got home. First we had to go all the way up to Lancashire to be 'demobbed', hand in our uniforms and be issued with 'demob' suits and the princely sum of £80. It was just over five years from the day I'd joined up: I was home and I had no regrets – save those concerning Ann and my little son.

As with most small hamlets, our village staged an annual fête: the first one since the war was held in Burnham Village soon after my discharge. There was always a funfair, coconut shies, plus all manner of 'try your skills' booths, and one that involved walking, blindfolded, for 10 paces before pulling on a piece of string so that it broke or released what was hanging above. At this event I won a pig.

My prize was probably about five or six months old, and I had to collect it from a local farmer who had donated it. The only transport I had was the motorbike I had bought with my demob money. My brother Edward and I drove up to the farm to discuss how we were going to get it home; but the farmer just picked up the pig, thrust it nose down in a back bag, handed it to my brother and bade us farewell.

So off we went with the pig thrashing about while being held over the shoulder of my pillion passenger. Halfway home it stopped jumping about; we got back, carried the pig to a sty we had built and laid it on the ground. But the pig did not move: it was dead, suffocated in the farmer's black bag.

The war might have been over, but Britain was still in the

grip of strict rationing. Under these regulations it was against the law to kill a pig below a certain weight: abattoirs were closely monitored to make sure the rules were stuck to.

But in Rhodesia I had learned to butcher a pig from watching a local farmer. I already knew how to prepare rabbit and deer – skills I had learned on my Scottish trip – so I proceeded to paunch the precious animal, with Mum running around supplying hot water to clear up the mess.

We then took the carcass over to our local abattoir where the man in charge asked who had butchered the pig. As he gave it a thorough examination I told him the whole story. But once he was done he turned to us and said: 'You've done a good job. There is nothing wrong with it, but I'm afraid you can't have any of it.' Since our pig had been killed illegally we were not allowed to have any our prize animal. Not even, as Mum put it, a sausage.

I spent the next week visiting old friends and catching up on what had been happening over the last five years. I discovered that 10 of my friends had not made it: killed in action, most of them RAF aircrew. I remember thinking that I had been lucky to fail my Morse code exam and be posted far away from all the action.

And my good fortune seemed to be continuing: I bumped into my old boss who promptly offered me my job back and also got me a £100 government grant to help me buy the tools I needed. I must say I felt a bit guilty about being so fortunate, but I picked up from where I had left off five years earlier.

It was some time after getting home, settling down and going back to work that I fell in love. Her name was Ann – which seemed to be something of a recurring theme – and she was still in the land army. Ann was from Wales and she sang and played the piano. I was then taking voice lessons and would happily practise my singing while she accompanied me. I saw her as often as I could: I took her home, introduced her to Mum and went all the way down to Wales to meet her family.

We talked about getting engaged. I was convinced I was in love – for the very first time – and I was besotted. Like me, Ann was no longer a virgin and I appreciated that on a number of occasions she wanted us to have sex. I didn't think of myself as old-fashioned but I convinced myself that we should wait: after all this was the woman I loved and she was a white girl, not like my previous conquests. No, Ann was to be the woman who would become my wife and, in accordance with the rules of society back then, I just knew that it was wrong to have sex before marriage. Not, of course, that we had set a date for the wedding: I had no money to speak of and we would have had nowhere to live.

First love can be such a cruel business. I discovered that Ann was going out with friends of mine on some of the days I was unable to see her: she went with them to dances and pubs and I was warned by a very close friend that she had had sex with one of the people I knew. I confronted her. We had a row, she admitted it and that was it: our love was broken – and along with it my heart.

Ann tried very hard to get me to forgive her, even going to see my mother to enlist her help. Mum did try, but for me that was it. I was very bitter and hurt, and maybe, too, there were other reasons why I could not countenance rekindling our love affair. It would be 14 more years before I touched another girl and she was the woman I took to be my wife:

on our wedding night she too was a virgin. But I wasn't – not by a long chalk. Not only had I stored up the experiences of Rhodesia and Mombasa, I had also spent a decade in a dangerous and illegal demi-monde. I had finally admitted to myself that I was gay – and I was hell-bent on making up for lost time.

FOUR

The first recorded mention of homosexuality in the laws of England was in 1300: it was not, as you might expect, a favourable notice.

Sex in all its forms has been particularly tied up with religion since the fall of the Roman Empire and the global rise of Christianity. Homosexuality was far from uncommon in Rome and, for a while at least, the early church didn't seem to have much of a problem, promoting a sex life that focused on fidelity and permanence in erotic relationships, pretty much regardless of who was doing what to whom. It was even common in the church's early days for homosexual unions to be performed.

But then around ad 400, Christianity began to introduce a new sexual code focused on the religious concepts of 'holiness' and 'purity'. Old Testament strictures against men loving men were resurrected until, by the Middle Ages, being attracted to the same sex could, and did, lead to brutally painful punishment.

In countries across Europe sex was permissible only within marriage and only when it was squarely aimed at procreation (and only then if the participants didn't enjoy it too much). Masturbation was out of bounds, as were anal and oral sex; all were devilishly pleasurable and did not lead to procreation.

In 13th-century France, for example, male homosexual behaviour resulted in castration on the first offence, dismemberment on the second, and burning on the third. Lesbian activity was punished with specific dismemberments for the first two offences and burning on the third. By the mid-14th century in many cities of Italy, laws against homosexuality were common and if a person was found to be homosexual, the city's government was entitled to confiscate the offender's property. By 1300, male homosexuality was a capital crime in more places than not.

Except for England. In medieval England such matters as 'unnatural sex' (as it was known) did not generally lead to prosecution in the King's courts; instead they were dealt with by priests hearing confession and who then imposed penances on the deviant soul in front of them. Then along came Henry.

The reign of Henry VIII was violent and repressive even by the standards of the time. The corpulent King formalised boiling to death as a suitable method of capital punishment, instituted the execution of the insane and – once he had split the Church of England from Rome and thus dispensed with the Canon Law which had been handling sexual 'offences' until then – made homosexuality a crime punishable by death. And death of a peculiarly vicious kind.

In 1533 Henry brought in a law that classified sodomy as an illegal act, whether it be between man and woman, man and man, or man and beast. (Was sexual activity between men and animals a major problem in Tudor England? History is silent on the subject – but evidently Henry felt it worthwhile to lump heterosexuals, homosexuals and medieval bestiality fans in the same outcast group.) And how was the miscreant to be executed? By being burned alive! Astonishingly, this law would stand, almost entirely unaltered, for more than 300 years.

It was not until 1869 that the Offences Against The Person Act abolished the death penalty for homosexuality, replacing it instead with a prison sentence that could range from 10 years to life. It also specified that for a prosecution to be brought, actual penetration had to be proven: oral sex, mutual masturbation, as well as other acts of non-penetration remained lawful. But if that sounds like a giant step forward, within 15 years the law once again turned nasty.

Henry Labouchère was the Liberal MP for Northampton. The Liberals were, at the time, the party of the rich and privileged and Mr Labouchère had founded a magazine that made its money by exposing 'moral degeneration'. He was particularly concerned by a supposed rise in homosexual activity. British society was then undergoing a great moral panic about homosexuality: Sir Howard Vincent, Scotland Yard's head of criminal investigations, had denounced it as 'a modern scourge', and one contemporary magazine, summed up the mood of the day with a trenchant editorial:

'The increase of these monsters in the shape of men, commonly designated margeries, poofs etc., of late years, in the great Metropolis, renders it necessary for the safety of the public that they should be made known... Will the reader credit it, but such is nevertheless the fact, that these monsters actually walk the street the same as the whores, looking out for a chance? Yes, the Quadrant, Fleet Street, Holborn, the Strand etc., are actually thronged with them! Nay, it is not long since, in the neighbourhood of Charing Cross, they posted bills in the windows of several public houses, cautioning the public to 'Beware of Sods!'

All of which encouraged Mr Labouchère to table – and get passed into law – an amendment to the 1885 Criminal Law Amendment Act by which 'gross indecency' between men would be punishable with a stiff prison sentence. Section 11 of the Act stated:

'Any male person who, in public or private, commits, or is a party to the commission of, or procures, or attempts to procure the commission by any male person of, any act of gross indecency with an other male person, shall be guilty of a misdemeanour, and being convicted thereof, shall be liable at the discretion of the Court to be imprisoned for any term not exceeding two years, with or without hard labour.'

The Labouchère Amendment, as it came to be known, never actually defined 'gross indecency' thereby allowing police the opportunity to arrest men for the previously noncriminal acts of mutual masturbation or oral sex. What's more, the new law made any sort of homosexual activity illegal even if it took place in private – and for good measure allowed for the prosecution of anyone who was 'party to the commission of' gross indecency, even if this meant it had taken place under their roof without their knowledge. A great many men would, in the decades to come, be ruined by this cruel piece of legislation. I would be one of them.

By the time I was born some of the worst of the moral panic had subsided. Gay men (not that we would have recognised the term) had begun to congregate in Britain's cities and had begun to form loose communities. Of course, local authorities and the police continued to harass them, but their efforts were often patchy. London, though, was a dangerous place to be homosexual: in the decade before I arrived into the world more than 100 men had been arrested, tried and imprisoned for the crime of being attracted to one another. And the figure would have been higher had it not been for a case which brought to the surface public disquiet over police methods – methods that I would come to know and have cause to fear before too long.

On 10 August 1927, a nationally known hero of World War One, Frank Champain, was sentenced to three months hard labour. Perhaps had it been anyone else, there things would have rested; but Champain appealed against his conviction and brought into the open the growing police practice of using *agents provocateurs*.

Champain was arrested in a public urinal by a detective who, in the space of 18 months, had caught and brought to court 12 homosexual men. His evidence in this latest case was that Champain had offered him a cigarette while standing at the stalls.

Now, it must be said that there is no doubt that Champain was gay and that he had visited a number of urinals already that day – and that the energetic policeman had been following him for an hour before the fatal offer of a smoke. But the case provoked a wave of disgust at the police tactics. The *Daily Mail* – never known for its sensitivity or tenderness – thundered: 'Here is a man who, because he offers a cigarette to a policeman in plain clothes, is hauled before a magistrate and is convicted.'

Champain won his appeal and the arrests of gay men in public toilets slowed to a trickle until the start of the 1930s. But then a new public panic set in, stoked by the Metropolitan Police and moral re-armament crusaders. Surveillance of public toilets was re-established, and from then until the outbreak of war more than 100 men every year were caught, tried and imprisoned for gross indecency.

But perhaps you're thinking that it served them right. After all, they were getting together for sex in public toilets. But read on, for it wasn't nearly as simple as it might now seem more than 70 years later.

Today, gay culture is well established in towns and cities throughout Britain, and the so-called gay pound is recognised as a reliable (and very welcome) source of income in these drab days of austerity. But at the time when I began to wonder whether I was one of the dreaded 'queers' or 'brown hatters' there was virtually nowhere for homosexual men to go. London was unusual in having anywhere at all – and even in the capital there were only a few clubs tucked discretely away in small side streets, usually on the first floor or in a basement, with plain and unmarked entrance doors. Unless you knew they were there, you would have walked past none the wiser.

The clubs were incredibly secretive, and for a very good reason. That Labouchère Amendment had made it a crime to be a party to homosexual behaviour of any sort – just hosting a meeting place for gay men was enough to risk prosecution. And so, even if you knew where to find a club, to become a member you had to be introduced and vouched for by an existing member. No one could just walk in off the street – after all, he might be an undercover policeman: it was members only, and everyone had to sign in on each visit.

The outcome of all this was 'cottaging'. A 'cottage' – so-called because many of them had, in those days, a pitched, tiled or thatched roof – is a public toilet, where men 'cruise' other men for sex. Today, of course, there are Internet sites dedicated to detailing exactly where the best cottages are to be found. But as I struggled with my sexuality in the late 1940s finding one depended on word of mouth and was an incredibly risky business.

Almost every week the papers would contain reports of those who had been caught, convicted and sent to prison. Added to that there was the very real danger of being beaten up by gay bashers – for, yes, they existed and were possibly even more ruthlessly brutal back then than their successors are today.

Given my emerging homosexual desires – spurred by memories of Mombasa – it was perhaps inevitable that I would discover cottaging. But as it happened I did so by accident. One day I was in a toilet in Slough, standing at the urinals and minding my own business, when a man came in, stood next to me, put his hand over and was about to catch hold of my penis. I was instinctively furious: he quickly realised the danger and ran out. I am sure in my own mind that if he hadn't I would have punched him.

But the incident played on my mind for some time. As a result I found myself back in this same toilet, hoping that it would happen again and knowing that if it did I would not hit anyone.

I want to be honest here. It is an absolute fact that, since homosexuality was illegal and rigorously punished, gay men (even emerging ones like me) could only get relief from their pent-up sexual energy by taking huge risks in public toilets. For highly sexed young men, quick, anonymous, uncomplicated sex in cottages was a very great – and vital – relief, dangerous or not.

But I have to admit that those very risks added to the thrill. Sex and adrenaline go well together and, before you know it, become addictive. And so I returned again and again to those public toilets in Slough: and it was in them that I met my very first gay friend: his name was Steven.

I don't think anything actually happened there. Nor did it later when, after speaking to Steven for some time, we went back to his sister's house. I remember that we just sat and talked. I was, of course, still very naïve: I had no real experience of actual sex with another man, but as we talked into the night I constantly remembered the young man in Mombasa. And I finally began to admit to myself that I might be bisexual or even fully homosexual. Strange as this thought was, I don't think I was greatly worried about what it might mean: I just knew that I wanted to meet someone – and that this someone would be a man. The question was: how?

Soon after my talk with Steven, I set out late one Saturday evening to go to London. I had heard that Piccadilly Circus was the place to go to find a man who would have sex with me. That this person would be doing so for money was, I confess, probably the least of my concerns. Most of my sexual experiences up until then had been with women who charged for sex. Since there was no real prospect of finding a male lover like myself (and indeed very great danger in trying to do so) I thought the thing to do was find a male prostitute.

I hadn't been there long before I was solicited by a young, good-looking man. He took me to a cheap hotel where we spent the night. I must have enjoyed what happened for early the next morning while we were both still in bed I told him I wanted to see him again. He agreed but he said he needed cigarettes and asked me to settle up with him: he promised that he would pop out to get fags and then come back to bed with me.

As he got to the door he looked back at me and asked, 'Do you trust me?' I was rather taken by surprise and instantly said, 'Yes'. He looked at me and asked if he could borrow my coat, as it was cold outside. And, naturally, I said, 'Okay'.

The minute that door closed I knew I had made a mistake – the first of many similar mistakes in my life. But I was naked and in bed; what could I do? I waited… and waited. But my first male lover never returned. When I finally trudged off home I was, perhaps, a little wiser than when I had come to London the previous night. I was unquestionably colder.

Despite what he had done I still wanted to see him again, and so one Saturday evening I set off for Piccadilly Circus once again. It was not difficult to find the young man: he was still wearing my coat. He was a little flustered and made some excuse for his behaviour. I looked at him and said, 'Okay, you can keep the coat, but can we go somewhere for a short time?'

This time I did not pay him until we were both about to leave the small hotel to which he had taken me. At that point I said, 'That session will cover the cost of the coat', quickly followed by 'Can I see you again?' He was somewhat disgruntled and did not seem too keen, but then he said, 'Yes, if you give me a fiver now.'

I took out a £5 note then started to tear it in half. He protested strongly, but I gave him half, said, 'See you' and walked off. The next time I saw him we went to a café and I bought him a coffee. As we were finishing it he suggested going to back to the little hotel together. But my heart wasn't in it. I said, 'No, I don't think so' – then gave him the other half of the £5 note and walked away.

I realised something that day, something which has stayed with me ever since. Casual sex was all well and good – and sometimes very good indeed – but I realised that except for men I fell in love with, the second time in bed with someone was never as good as the first.

Perhaps you are now looking at me in a new light: disturbed, maybe, by what you are reading. After all, I had willingly had sex with prostitutes – male or female – and picking up a rent boy (as young men on the game were euphemistically known) is hardly the stuff of romance. Well, you are not alone. During this time I fought a great deal with my conscience, resolving to stop what I was doing, change the way I was thinking and what I was thinking about.

It has to be remembered that back then there was no help whatsoever for homosexuals. There was nothing in print, excepting the harsh statute laws prohibiting our love and the vicious newspaper articles that followed our arrest and/or prosecutions. The only media was the BBC – and ironically, given what we now know about many of its stars, there was never anything on the wireless or television about being gay. And at a time when most people had shared telephone 'party' lines (if they had a phone at all), the notion of a telephone helpline was light years away.

On a personal basis I had only my one gay friend, Steven, and a few acquaintances – others like him – that I had now met. But they were no help at all towards my angst and uncertainty because they had not only accepted the way they were but seemed very happy about it.

I had resolved to go and see our family doctor, and so one day I went nervously to his surgery. There were only a couple of patients in the waiting room: the first was in and out in a short time, and I moved up in the queue. But by the time the next patient had been in with the doctor for 20 minutes I suddenly got up and rushed out.

I realised that opening up to the doctor would have been a huge and very dangerous mistake. Dr Summers was the epitome of a red-blooded British army colonel – a very large man with a loud voice and an Eton College accent. He was, I think, about as heterosexual as any man alive.

He was also close to, and fond of, my mother and family. What would he have said if I'd told him that I was sexually aroused by other men, let alone that I had been to bed with a male prostitute? Don't forget that not only was the NHS less than a year old at the time, but that I would also have been confessing to a serious criminal offence. What sort of position would that have put him in? Would he have reported me – perhaps feeling he was obliged to report me – to the police? At best he would probably have brusquely told me to pull myself together. He would probably have addressed me as 'my boy', would have asked with incredulity what my mother would think if she knew, and then told me to grow up and get out of his surgery.

I tried from then on to bury myself in my work and dismiss my terrible secret. I resolved to be on the go from seven in the morning till midnight seven days a week and (a word I would come to know very well) to sublimate my desires.

But then, in some of us the sex drive is very strong. Looking back I realise that I have always been addicted to sex. Those addicted to tobacco, drink, drugs or gambling (which unlike the above are self-inflicted and can be cured) will know what I mean when I say that once hooked, always hooked. And so, despite my best intentions, I started to mix more and more with men who (I reluctantly admitted to myself) were made the same way as me. But in a feeble attempt to keep at least part of my resolution intact, I did so only on a Saturday evening.

There was, at that time, a pub in Windsor called The Ship. This was where 'men who went with men' (as it was dismissively described in those days) would meet. Most were ordinary men burdened by a love that was still illegal; some though were like the young man from Piccadilly Circus – prostitutes who had sex for money. Some of these were members of the local army guardsmen stationed at Windsor Castle.

And so, one evening, I casually told my father (himself a former guardsman who had been based there) that I was going into Windsor for a drink. For almost 70 years I have remembered what he said: 'Steer clear of The Ship, son – that's where the queers go.' I wondered had he guessed? He never said anything further – and I would not open up to him until almost 25 years had passed.

But Dad was right: The Ship *was* where queers went. I was one of them – and I was about to start living a double life.

FIVE

The year was 1949. I was 26 years old. I had been overseas in the service of my country. I had lost my heterosexual and homosexual virginity – and knew which event I found more fulfilling. I was a tall, good-looking gay man who had resolved to marry an innocent (for which read virginal) woman; and I was spending my Saturday evenings in the company of a cast of outlaws who, like me, were risking everything for their desires. Many were, again like me, leading double lives and probably (I certainly was) doing their level best to subsume their homosexuality in the day-to-day austerity of post-war work and society.

My chosen sublimations were singing, the Scouts and my chosen profession as a patternmaker. Unfortunately I was about to get the sack.

I was by then what was called a journeyman: a fully

qualified craftsman at Wagstaff's, the only pattern shop in the Slough area. We were constantly very busy, servicing a large number of foundries on the local trading estate. We rarely did fewer than 60 hours a week – the official working week in those days being 48 hours, with overtime on Saturday mornings and evenings.

I had a couple of friends who were starting up their own business in a garden shed: they asked me if I could make them a few small patterns. They said that my employers were very expensive and Mr Wagstaff's deliveries took too long. Without giving it too much thought as to what I was doing, I said I would. As far as I was concerned it meant that I would be working for a few hours extra – until at least midnight every day, Saturday afternoons and Sundays – and more importantly working without any machinery or many of the specialist tools of my trade.

I had been in the Scout movement since my return from the war. And being a good Boy Scout I stole absolutely nothing from work: not wood, not screws, glue or pattern paint. Not even time, for I did this outside our working hours. Frankly, I think I would have been quite justified in taking a bit of something, since I had discovered from the office staff that Mr Wagstaff had been paying me short from the money that the government gave him to make up my wages. But no: I was a Scout – and stealing anything was utterly outside the Scouting code.

When I had finished the equipment that my friends needed, they took them to one of the local foundries to be cast. Mr Wagstaff, who called at all of these factories in the course of his day-to-day business, saw them, and found out that I had made them. He sacked me on the spot.

I was devastated: the next nearest pattern shop was in Reading, 15 miles away. In those days, for them to consider me I would have had to have a reference: there was no possibility of Mr Wagstaff providing me with anything but a damning account of my 'treachery' and I was absolutely sure they wouldn't employ me if they were told what I had done. I went home early, utterly disconsolate and with a face like a wet weekend in Scarborough. Mum knew straight away that something was wrong, but I couldn't bring myself to tell her. Then in the evening there was a knock on the door: it was someone I had seen many times in the pattern shop – an important customer of Mr Wagstaff's who owned an aluminium foundry in nearby Cippenham. He had been told what had happened and had come to see me with a proposal.

He said it was about time there was some competition in the local pattern trade. He denounced Mr Wagstaff for having a monopoly, for over-charging and for being late with deliveries. If I were to set up on my own, he would give me as much work as I could handle. I don't actually remember what I said to this man who was throwing me a lifeline: I must have said yes, but when he had gone reality set in. How could I set up as a patternmaker? I had no workshop, no machinery and no capital. Frankly, if there had been another pattern shop near I would have gone there and positively begged for a job.

But that, of course, was rather the point. There wasn't: which meant I had no choice but to start my own business. It was a daunting prospect; I had left school with no real qualifications, and being self-employed – let alone running my own industrial business – had never ever crossed my mind. But there's my luck again: it was fortunate (as it turned out) that there was no alternative. And so I spent my savings, borrowed some money from Mum, cleaned out a corner of Dad's coal shed, scrounged some scrap castings, made a treadle lathe out of an old treadle sewing machine… and got started.

I had no electricity or gaslight, only a Tilley lamp for which the paraffin fuel had to be pumped up by hand. Since a great deal of patternmaking usually needs specialist machinery and electric hand tools, everything took me twice as long to make as it would have had I been in a pattern shop like Wagstaff's.

And of course I also had to do all of the running around that Mr Wagstaff had handled: quoting on jobs as well as delivering everything on my motorbike. And after all that I discovered the downside of running your own business: nobody pays their bills for at least six weeks, often ten. I ran up a debt on my housekeeping with Mum and spent no money at all on myself for weeks.

I was working 14 hours a day; I had no social life and no time to devote to the sport I had come to love: squash. But there was an upside to all this: it took my mind off sex – I simply didn't have a spare moment to worry about my desires, let alone pursue them.

After about six months I found a man who had a fair-sized workshop in his garden and from which he had been running a small business. He had fallen ill with tuberculosis, a serious problem in those days, and was unable to work while convalescing. We came to an arrangement whereby I rented his workshop from him. And – joy of joys! – it had electricity.

But how to finance this modest expansion of my little business? For the first time in my life, and with considerable fear and trepidation, I made an appointment to see the local bank manager: I fully expected my request for an overdraft to be turned down. To my delight he offered me more than I requested. What I didn't realise as I walked out of his office was how difficult it would be to pay off the loan as well as the interest. From that day forward I was to be saddled with an overdraft for most of the next 47 years.

Eventually my landlord recovered from TB and needed his workshop back. Eventually I found a proper builders' workshop which was quite large and that had everything I needed: three-phase electricity and a lot of medium-sized woodworking machinery, with an old-fashioned 'tortoise' stove in the centre, just like the one in the laundry at home. In the summer we could save the scrap wood and shavings – which could be burned in the winter to give us free heat. My fledging enterprise was finally on a sound footing and my life seemed to be on the up and up.

Fate has a funny way of tripping you up. It has happened to me time and time again; just when things seem to be going well life has a habit of getting in the way. And yet after Christmas 1949 it wasn't life that caused the trouble: it was death.

I was down at the works. In those days there was less of a tradition of taking time off between Christmas and New Year. The phone rang. It was the police telling me that my brother Edward had been involved in an accident.

I rushed home to find Mum in a flood of tears. A policeman was there too. He told me that Edward had been returning from the pub, riding pillion on a friend's motorbike and they had collided with a lorry. My brother was dead.

Apparently, Edward and his friend had been in the pub for a lunchtime drink. There was no suggestion that they had had too much to drink – though since there was no such thing as a breathalyser back then it would have been impossible to tell in any event. Unfortunately neither were crash helmets compulsory in those days: had Edward been wearing one, I'm sure he would have survived.

I went with the policeman to identify my brother's body. On the way back from the hospital we stopped at the crash scene. It was on a T-junction, very close to home. On the last left-hand bend they must have taken it a bit too fast and too wide. A lorry going the other way and turning left swung out to take the tight corner and they met head on. My brother had been thrown though the air and his head struck the tall garden wall of a nearby house. I discovered a small tuft of Edward's hair on the wall.

It took a very long time to get over this. It was most difficult for Mum, partly I think because he was always a little on the delicate side and because she had fought so long and hard to keep him alive when he was so ill as a baby. She said simply: 'To lose him like this, after all we went through.' He was just 23 years old.

I was, of course, still wildly conflicted about my sexuality and suffering – when time and emotions permitted – terrible worries about the tension between my desires and what was considered acceptable (or even legal) by society. Happily, though, I had something else to divert my thoughts – two passions that were to be with me for the next quarter of a century.

I had joined the local church choir at the tender age of seven, largely, as I said earlier, to cure my terrible stammer. Once a year we would take part in a Choir Festival. For a few weeks beforehand we would rehearse several pieces of special music, then on the big day we would all go to St George's Chapel, Windsor Castle, where there would be many other choirs including the St George's Choir and the Eton College Choir. There were so many of us that we filled more than half the Chapel.

A rehearsal was held first. Then we would have half an hour's break before putting on our cassocks and surplices that we'd previously taken home to be washed and ironed. Being a professional laundress, mum would put some starch on my surplice. I thought it always looked the best. We then processed right round the chapel and up the steps, just like the Knights of the Garter do. I think, perhaps, that in the dressing up and performing were planted the seeds of something which would, nearly 20 years later, come to dominate my life – and would both bring immense pleasure and, eventually, terrible pain.

Our parents and members of the public were invited to the Festival. We very much enjoyed the sound of this mass choir in the magnificent surroundings of St George's Chapel, where the acoustics were perfect. It always inspired me to sing my best. There were always several solos for which there was an audition. I decided that one day I would audition.

I sang my first solo at eight and a half years old – a verse from *Away in a Manger* during a carol service. From then on I often performed solos, not only at the church services but also at weddings and funerals. I was also put forward for the audition at St George's Chapel. There were nine boys competing, and though I was not successful that time, I was chosen the next year and the year after that.

My voice didn't break until I was nearly 16. When you are as interested as I was in singing as a boy, you wonder what voice you will have when it does break. I did experiment with my range and was a bit disappointed when I knew I would be a bass or a baritone. I dearly wanted to be a tenor – tenors are always the most popular: they have most of the best music written for them and are always the most popular and in great demand. Still, a voice is what it is and I joined as a bass-baritone. I discovered that I had a very good range: a bass or baritone voice can also sing in falsetto.

In the RAF I would often sing in the canteens (but only after I had a few beers). *Ave Maria* was all the rage at that time and I would sometimes sing this in alto. The boys would cheer and tell me to drop my trousers to prove I was a male.

The very first Sunday I was home after the war I visited the church again, but was very disappointed at what I found. The choirmaster I had known had left, there were hardly any boys in the choir and no men. I did what I could, but the old Vicar had died; the new one was not very interested in the choir and was talking of having girls to make up the numbers. For me that was the last straw. Fortunately, I was head hunted by Burnham Church, where there was a very good choir: it was a move that led me – via a meeting with a very talented pianist – to consider a career as a professional singer.

For a time I did professional engagements for annual dinners such as Masonic Lodges and ex-servicemen's associations. But at times I found it difficult to accept the life of a professional singer. I usually performed after the dinner, by which times the audience had enjoyed a few drinks. On one occasion they were rowdy and insisted on chatting away throughout my songs. After a while I'd had enough – I stopped mid-note, walked off the stage and told them to keep the fee.

This experience led me to assess my prospects and to realise that I had been born too late. Fifty years earlier I might have been able to make a go of singing as a career. But television was coming in fast and these were the days of Cliff Richard, Adam Faith and Tommy Steele: the sort of music that I sang was getting less and less popular, especially with young people. And after that bad experience I knew that I only wanted to sing to those who actually wanted to listen to me.

If that makes me sound a bit of a prima donna, I apologise. But, as things turned out, there was another outlet for my singing – and one that helped other people as well as allowing me to open my mouth.

I had joined the Wolf Cubs of my local Scout group at the age of nine. After I graduated to the full pack, Scouting became an integral part of my life. It's not particularly fashionable to say this now, but I – and a great many other men – owe a huge amount to the people who gave up their time to run these packs. It was Ralph Reader – the singer and theatrical producer whose name would forever be linked with all the best aspects of Scouting – who put it best:

'To be commended are those who are not only mindful of the rightful upbringing of their own, but also of other men's sons.'

Today, television, the Internet and a weakening of the communal sprit of responsibility has, in my view, led to a lack of good leaders and role models for the most important age group of growing boys or young men. The ages of 12 to 18, are vital years, and in the past Scouting played an enormously important role in helping youngsters grow from childhood into responsible adults. Sadly, we now see many groups closing for lack of leaders – as well as others suffering because of a shortage of leaders of the right quality.

During my pre-war Scouting days my troop put on three Gang Shows. For those not familiar with the term, Gang Shows were a Scouting phenomenon. In 1931 Ralph Reader was asked to write an amateur variety show to raise money for a Scout camp. Reader put together a mixture of song, dance and short comedy sketches. Some were stand-alone items; others were a series of songs on a chosen theme, or a running gag. Initially the show did not have a title, but during a rehearsal break Reader asked a cast member if everyone was ready, to which the response was: 'Aye-aye, Skip, the gang's all here.' That line struck an immediate chord and the first Gang show production ran for more than a month at a prestigious West End theatre in the winter of 1932.

Although not all of the performances sold out, the show easily hit its fundraising target and Baden-Powell – the founder and head of the worldwide Scout movement – asked Reader to produce it again the following year. A tradition was established and within six years of Reader first putting pen to paper the London Gang Show achieved the distinction of being the first amateur production to have a Royal Command Performance.

Now, the 'London Gang Show' was the pinnacle

performance. However, Scouts all over the world put on local Gang Shows in their own neighbourhoods every year. The war put an end to all such performances, but after I was demobbed I had rejoined the Scouting movement as a local leader and, before long, it was decided to put on a district Gang Show. I was put forward as the producer because of my singing: reluctantly I agreed. Little did I know then how much of my life would be consumed by this – nor how it would, in time, come to haunt me.

We put on two shows and a matinee making the princely profit of £30 – no small sum in 1949. We then had a request to take the show up to the local hospital run by the Canadian Red Cross in the grounds of Lord and Lady Astor's estate at Cliveden, Taplow. The first four wards were a special unit for the research on rheumatism in children. Wards 1 and 2 were for boys and girls aged up to 12 years. Ward 3 was for girls 12 to 18 years and ward 4 was for boys 12 to 18. Each ward was full, with some 36 beds in each.

The show was staged in the small hospital theatre. We played to an audience made up mostly of the older children who were well enough to attend from the unit, some still in their beds, some sitting on the beds and some in wheelchairs. A few of the boys were wearing odd bits of Scout uniform, and when the show was over we talked to these boys while taking them back to their wards. They told us that there had been a Scoutmaster who used run a meeting in Ward 4, but that he had stopped coming some time ago.

At the next meeting of our local Scouting association I mentioned this, pointing out that we ought to do something about getting things going again. The result was that I was handed a Scoutmaster's warrant and told to get on with it.

My first task was to learn as much as I could about the conditions that had brought these lads to this special unit. I discovered that rheumatic fever can severely damage the valves of the heart and was caused mainly by neglect or poor social conditions. I also discovered that many of the boys were so disabled that they could not feed themselves.

At the first meeting, there were 36 boys in the ward. They came from all over the South of England, and from very different backgrounds: one had been sent from Borstal – the youth prison system – and one from Eton College. The job of feeding them was very time-consuming for the nurses – and so it was one of the first tasks our new troop got stuck into. Right away we became popular with the nurses and the Ward Sister. They, along with the doctors, realised that Scouting was therapeutic for their patients. Boys were there for a minimum of three months, most for much longer, many for several years.

At the time I was no more than six months into my business venture. At first I wondered if I had taken on too much, but soon realised what I came to be very certain of – and continued to be certain of for the next 25 years – that if you do something right and important, the more you put into it the more satisfaction, peace of mind and downright enjoyment you get out of it.

Most of the boys I worked with would never be fit and well, some would not live to reach adulthood. How could I, as fit and healthy as it was possible to be, with seemingly boundless energy, not do what I could to make the lives of these lads a little brighter?

I would walk into the ward and 30 smiling faces would look up and shout, "Ello Skip'. My tiredness and worries would drop away almost instantly, my cares and problems were nothing compared to theirs. I was constantly in awe of their cheerfulness, their zest for life and the acceptance of their lot: they had a lot to complain about, but never once did.

For those who improved to point of being able to sit up and to feed themselves there was very little of the Scout training programme that could not be carried out – and what couldn't be accomplished easily we somehow improvised. We constructed a special tray to enable them to do the fire-lighting test on the bed in front of them, and we had an altar fire made out of welded steel with a spit so that they could cook from their bed. They enjoyed stoking the fire and turning the handle. And if the other lads enjoyed the meal a boy had cooked, well then he'd passed his cooking test.

Pioneering was done in miniature. They particularly enjoyed the knots, and I put in fun ones such as the highwayman's hitch, the hangman's noose and the thief knot. They learned surprisingly quickly, probably quicker than most in an able-bodied troop seeing that they were all together all of the time. And time, of course, was something they had plenty of.

Many of the lads came from deprived backgrounds and some from many miles away so they often had no visitors. Sunday was the only visiting day. After a while we had a word with the parents that did come to visit: with their blessing my assistants and I either sat with those that had no one coming to see them, or took those who could manage it out on trips.

At Christmas the whole ward was transformed, with a different theme each year. Extra visiting days were allowed and we made sure that those without a visitor had one from a special group of supporters set up to help in all the ways that a parents' association would do for an able-bodied group.

Gradually, and almost without me realising it, Scouting became a vocation and almost an obsession. For several hours every day, often until the early hours, I would be planning, writing letters, telephoning – doing everything and anything to give something to the organisation I loved and the lads who joined our troops. Looking back I can now see that for me Scouting was sublimation, for I had not come to terms with my sexuality.

We need to be careful here. In our modern world there is immense suspicion about men who give up their free time to devote themselves to running Scout troops. In the late 1940s and early 1950s, despite the fact that homosexuality was illegal and gay men were persecuted for their desires, there was much less of an understanding of the fact that some – and I repeat, some – of them do so for ulterior motives.

Some time ago I saw the film about the life of Baden-Powell. I was not surprised – and nor was I in disagreement – at the suggestion made in the programme that he probably had problems with his sexuality. In fact, had he not had iron self-control, then I think he would probably have been an active paedophile. When, as a young military officer, he was shown a picture of a number of naked pre-pubertal boys he asked if he could have a copy. And from the outset of the movement, at his first Scout camp, all the boys had a somewhat telling morning ritual to perform. Baden-Powell instructed them to form a circle, completely naked and, having picked up a container full of cold water, they were

GEORGE MONTAGUE

given B-P's signal to tip the container of water over the boy in front of them. Baden-Powell called this odd-sounding procedure 'Kippers'.

Now, I have never been sexually attracted to boys, but from the earliest days of my involvement in the movement I was very well aware that Scouting is a very big attraction to those who are. I even had some doubt about the sexuality of some of my adult unmarried male helpers, and so – without letting anyone else know – I kept a close eye on them.

Paedophilia and homosexuality are two very different things. I was a gay man – albeit one struggling to come to terms with his feelings and desires – but I was not a paedophile. Unfortunately, not everyone can – or could – see the difference. And, though I could not have known it back then, the climate of public hostility to homosexuality would one day claim me as a victim.

SIX

Alan Mathison Turing was one of the greatest minds this country has ever produced. A brilliant mathematician, he was one of the most influential figures in the development of computer science and – most crucially – during World War Two he invented the Colossus machine at Bletchley Park which broke the secrets of the Enigma codes of German U-boats in the Atlantic.

Turing's work shortened the Second World War by two years, saving hundreds of thousands of lives, and preventing starvation throughout Britain by revealing the location of U-Boats that were intercepting merchant ships.

But on 7 June 1954, he committed suicide by biting into a poisoned apple. Alan Turing was gay; he was also a victim of the law.

The 1950s were a time of great social change in Britain. At

the end of the war, Churchill – the great leader who had come to symbolise our fight against the evil of Nazi Germany – was unceremoniously dumped out of office in a general election fought on the novel basis of a fairer deal for ordinary people. The sea change in British political life brought in the welfare state and the National Health Service – and an understanding that the stuffy, self-satisfied conservatism of the past was being swept away.

But was it really?

As far as attitudes to homosexuality were concerned, British society – at least in so far as it was represented in Parliament, the Courts and the attitudes of the police – was becoming more intolerant, not less.

Anti-gay persecution had been building for some time. In the 15 years following the outbreak of World War Two, the number of recorded indictable homosexual offences increased dramatically. In 1938, the police in England and Wales dealt with 134 cases of sodomy; in 1952, that figure has risen to 670; by 1954, it was 1,043. By the following year, there were 2,322 recorded instances of 'gross indecency' in England and Wales, compared with 316 in 1938.

In the early days of the war there had been some degree of tolerance within the ranks for casual same-sex acts – as long, of course, as there was no explicit claiming of a homosexual identity. But, as the years wore on, military authorities became increasingly concerned about homosexual activities. During the first 12 months of the war, 48 serving men were court-martialled for 'indecency between males'; five years later, in the final 12 months between 1944 and 1945, the number of court martials for homosexual acts had increased to 324. It is an astonishing fact that over the entire duration of the war, there were more British men court-martialled for homosexual acts than for any other category of offence.

And justice, if that's what you can call it, was harsh. Sir Paul Latham was a wealthy Conservative MP. Although he had been exempted from military service, he volunteered anyway and joined the army to fight for his country. But in 1941, he was tried and convicted of 'improper behaviour' with three gunners and a civilian while serving as an officer in the Royal Artillery. He was convicted of 10 charges of indecent conduct, discharged dishonourably, imprisoned for two years, and forced to resign his seat in Parliament.

Whenever I hear of cases like Latham's I remember a powerful statement by a US Army veteran, Leonard Matlovich:

'When I was in the military they gave me a medal for killing two men – and a discharge for loving one.'

During the course of the war, newspapers increasingly featured stories claiming that military personnel stationed in British communities were in danger of corruption by predatory homosexuals. And nor was this simply a tabloid frenzy: in wartime Britain newspapers were subject to strict censorship as well as being desperately short of paper. If these stories made it into the press, then it's a fair bet that they did so with – at the very least – the blessing of the government.

And in response to the public outcry incited by these accounts, police forces started to utilise the Defence Regulations and Emergency Powers Acts to close 'disorderly' premises without following the required legal procedures.

There were few enough places for gay men to meet: now

the police began targeting them. In 1941 Sam's Café in Rupert Street, London, was – under the dubious authority of this Act – closed between the hours of 6pm and 6am. Three years later several prominent gay-friendly pubs were formally cautioned for harbouring 'sodomites'. As the police bore down, many pubs and cafés which had turned a blind eye to homosexual patrons voluntarily began to exclude them – if only to avoid being harassed by the police.

The growing persecution of homosexuals coincided with the appointment in 1944 of Sir Theobald Mathew as Director of Public Prosecution (a post he would go on to hold for another 22 years). Mathew was horrified by the recorded increase in homosexual incidents during the war years, and officially made the suppression of homosexuality a top priority.

Local police authorities – the bodies of the great and good who decided policy in their area – introduced specific targets for the arrest of homosexual men. And to ensure these targets were met they devised a set of procedures by which gays might be caught. By the late 1940s, the Metropolitan Police in London was even offering detailed training courses and teaching officers how to go 'underground' in homosexual milieus. Entrapment became common, and men were often arrested after performing sexual acts with policemen.

Then, in 1951, it got even worse. Two British secret service agents, Guy Burgess and Donald Maclean, defected to the Soviet Union. Both were revealed to be homosexuals. In the outburst of public hand-wringing that followed, the idea that 'sexual deviance' was detrimental to the well-being of the nation took a firm hold. The British government began searching for, and weeding out, homosexuals in sensitive government positions.

It was in the midst of this atmosphere of moral panic that Alan Turing was arrested. In January 1952, Turing had started a relationship with Arnold Murray, a 19-year-old unemployed man. Turing had met Murray just before Christmas outside the Regal Cinema in Manchester's Oxford Road, and had invited him to lunch. On 23 January Turing's house was burgled and Murray told Turing that he knew who the burglar was. Turing reported the crime to the police and, in honestly answering their questions, he said that he was having a sexual relationship with Murray. The police then promptly arrested both of them, and charged them under Section 11 of the Criminal Law Amendment Act – the old Labouchère Amendment.

On 27 February, Turing was arraigned in court as part of the committal proceedings. He reserved his defence, neither claiming to be innocent nor admitting his guilt. But by the time the case came to trial, on 31 March 1952, his lawyers had persuaded him to plead guilty – despite the fact that he felt no remorse or guilt for having committed homosexual acts. He was convicted and given a choice between imprisonment or probation conditional on his agreement to undergo chemical castration. Turing accepted the option of treatment and was prescribed injections of a synthetic oestrogen, which lasted a full year. The drugs rendered him completely impotent.

Turing's conviction led to the removal of his security clearance, and thus robbed the British government of one of its most brilliant scientists at a time when science was vital to the country's national interest. For good measure, the conviction meant that Turing was also denied entry into the United States.

Not surprisingly, Turing became depressed – not least because the court-imposed treatment caused him to grow breasts. On 8 June 1954, Turing's cleaner found him dead. He had died the previous day from cyanide poisoning. A half-eaten apple lay beside his bed: this was how he had ingested the drug that killed him.

It would be almost 60 years before the British government apologised for the prosecution of one of its most brilliant and important scientists: in 2013 he received a Parliamentary pardon.

The years immediately following Turing's arrest saw an ever-greater crackdown on gay men. Emboldened by a public mood of intense homophobia, police began to prosecute prominent figures for homosexual acts and indecent behaviour. By 1953 there were more than 10,000 gay arrests a year, including three prominent MPs and a succession of actors. Of these, the best known was Sir John Gielgud. Shortly after he was knighted in 1953, Gielgud was in rehearsals for a West End play. After drinks one evening he decided to visit one of London's cottages – an underground public lavatory – to seek out a gay lover.

He had done this many times before, but this time he was arrested by Scotland Yard's so-called 'Pretty Police' – young recruits picked for their looks and stationed in the urinals for the purposes of entrapment – and charged with 'persistently importuning men for immoral purposes'. He was fined £10 and advised to see a doctor to 'cure' his unnatural desires. A reporter for the *London Evening Standard* happened to be in court and Gielgud's conviction was splashed over the afternoon editions. Gielgud, a sensitive soul at the best of times, was humiliated, and the situation was made even worse when a Conservative peer called for him to be horsewhipped in the street after being stripped of his knighthood.

In some ways Gielgud got off lightly – perhaps because of the very celebrity that ensured the unwelcome headlines. Many other less famous men were given much more severe punishment. The treatment of Rupert Croft-Cooke – an author and, like me, a man who had served his country in World War Two – was all too typical. Cooke's secretary and companion, Joseph Alexander, had met two Royal Navy cooks in the Fitzroy Tavern, one of the few gay-friendly pubs in London's West End at that time. Alexander invited them to spend the weekend at Croft-Cooke's house in East Sussex.

During the weekend, they both – quite willingly – had sex with Alexander and Croft-Cooke. But on their way home from the weekend, they got drunk and assaulted two men, one of whom was a policeman. They were arrested, but the police were more interested in what they had been doing during the weekend. In the end, and to get immunity from prosecution for the assault charges, both sailors gave statements about having sex with Croft-Cooke. The author was duly arrested, tried and sent to prison for nine months. It was a dramatic demonstration that homosexuals weren't safe, even in their own homes. It would not be the last such demonstration.

The police and the government were dedicated to stamping out what they saw as the 'homosexual menace' in society, whatever the cost. But we are all human and all have our needs, so gay men, myself included, continued to face the risk of arrest and imprisonment. Clubs and pubs that allowed us to meet were themselves running the risk of prosecution: perhaps that explains why there were so few of them – as well as the febrile ambiance inside them (unlike anything that exists today, I'm sorry to say).

I've been trying to find the right phrase to describe this: the best I can come up with is an atmosphere of relaxed gaiety. And in writing this down I have just this second realised that perhaps this is why we eventually called ourselves gay. And, looking back, I see that there was an inherent contradiction in the mood inside these clubs and bars: it was both totally relaxed and happy, yet simultaneously it pulsed with a sort of electricity.

So what sort of people were we – homosexual men in an era when to be gay was to be a criminal? We were all sorts, that's what. There were a few very camp men (and I must tell you now that I vowed never to act in that way) who would literally and metaphorically let their hair down. But the rest of us must have looked like the rest of British society outside: dull and rather drab.

The reason, of course, was that almost everyone there, even the effeminate ones, were what we would now call 'in the closet': they – we – were leading double lives, keeping secrets from their families and denied by law the fundamental right of setting up home with a partner.

The clubs were only open until 11 o'clock of an evening, so we would arrange bottle parties. There were always several being arranged: all I had to do was decide which one to go to. At these parties I would invariably meet someone about my own age, go home with him, arrange to meet again, think about him all week, then meet him again on the following Saturday. But Montague's Law applied every time: the second time with a lover was never the same.

Does this make me sound promiscuous? Promiscuity is one of the things gay men have been, and still are, condemned for. To be homosexual is, according to this way of thinking, to be promiscuous. But I honestly believe that as a general rule it's a fallacy: many heterosexual people are just as – often more – promiscuous: they have one-night stands and longer term affairs just as we do. And for decades now there have been swingers clubs where every weekend thousands of straight couples meet and have sex with complete strangers. Is this really any different from the gay scene? And although heterosexual couples have a great many more reasons and pressures to stay married – children being the most obvious – divorce is endemic. I know many male couples that have been together all their adult lives: so much for promiscuity and homosexuality always going hand in hand.

In any event, my excursions were rare oases of pleasure in an otherwise hectic schedule of Scouting and work. My business was growing and since my customers were spread out all over the south of England I spent many hours driving around the countryside.

Good patternmakers were like gold dust in those days and never unemployed, and so I had to take on apprentices and train them. This, I think, was one of the main reasons for the success of my growing business. I advertised in the local press and gave details to the local youth employment office once a year. By chance, the youth employment officer that I saw was the very same one that I had seen all those years before when I was 14. He helped me a lot by vetting the boys himself and only sending me the most likely candidates.

I began a deliberate strategy whereby I took on one apprentice every year. I would interview four or five, then

I would visit the home of each one, talk to the parents, telling them that if their son was chosen he would find patternmaking a very exacting craft and it would be a long time before he would be able to call himself a patternmaker. I stressed that both he and I would need their support. It was also important to me what their hobbies were and, of course, how they had done at school. And so I visited the headmaster and the woodwork teacher. It all added to the miles I drove each year, but I found it paid dividends, for I was choosing only those that would lay the golden eggs for the company. And, as the years rolled on, I had very few failures. Most of my apprentices stayed for many years and, even if they left, they often returned to rejoin our company.

My duties with the Scouts were also absorbing huge amounts of time and energy. In the summer of 1951, the government organised the Festival of Britain – a showcase for the country (and the world) to promote science, technology, industrial design, architecture and the arts. The abiding symbol of the whole affair was The Skylon – a futuristic cigar-shaped structure of metal latticework which was supported on cables, but which actually appeared to float 50 feet off the ground on London's South Bank.

My Scouts were, of course, unable to get out of the hospital to see this modern wonder for themselves – so we built a our own model Skylon in the hospital ward. On another occasion a working model railway ran down the centre of the ward. For the Queen's Coronation in June 1953 we produced a newsletter – the first edition of many that would follow. Inevitably it had a picture of Her Majesty on the front, but inside it featured contributions by the boys themselves. What was more, they printed it themselves in the ward on an old duplicator.

We had by now become a formal Scout Group – a designation that comes only with clear size and support. We had approximately 30 Wolf Cubs in Wards 1 and 2, and before very long, with a few hints and a bit of help, packs of Brownies were set up on the same wards, followed by Girl Guides in Ward 3. Guy Fawkes Night was one of the highlights of the year. There was a large grass area at the back of the wards and beyond that a wood, so we were able to build a real fire complete with a Guy Fawkes, made, naturally, by the Cubs, Scouts, Brownies and Guides themselves.

I like to think that the work we adults put in was helping much more than the morale of the boys and girls stuck on the wards. Certainly, the length of the average stay was very much reduced – down sometimes from several years to several months.

But rheumatic fever was a nasty illness: it could severely damage a child's heart, and since more and more strain was put on this as they got older, quite a number of these young people never reached adulthood. At least five died at the hospital during my time there, including one who was our Troop Leader when he died at the age of just 17 years. Brian Walker was his name and he was with us for over three years: I had given him my nomination for the award of the Cornwell Scout Badge – an award for outstanding fortitude and bravery, named after a 15-year-old boy sailor who died in the battle of Jutland in the World War One. It is one of my great sorrows that Brian died before it could be presented.

I was 30 years old now and working all the hours God

sent on my growing business, devoting all the spare time I could find to the Scouts – and somehow combining all this with my secret double life in the exciting and perilous demimonde of 1950s homosexuality. I was also still living at home with Mum and Dad.

But in the summer of 1953 two great events would change my world. The first was instantaneously positive; the second truly frightening.

SEVEN

On Friday, 16 October 1953, the Metropolitan Police announced the arrest of Lord Edward Montagu and his friend film director Kenneth Hume for 'serious offences' with Boy Scouts. The news provoked a frenzy of media coverage.

Lord Montagu – or, to give him his full and proper title, the Third Baron Montagu of Beaulieu in the County of Hampshire – was then a 28-year-old socialite and the youngest peer in the House of Lords. His arrest, and subsequently his appearance before Winchester Assizes, set the country alight: here was a Peer of the Realm – one of the pillars of British society facing terrible allegations that he had sexually molested a 14-year-old Boy Scout at a beach hut on the Solent. It mattered little that Lord Montagu denied the charge: the mere suggestion that such a high-born, and high-profile, member of the aristocracy might be a homosexual – and an apparently predatory one at that – played into the growing political consensus that 'something must be done'.

The then Home Secretary, Sir David Maxwell Fyfe, had promised 'a new drive against male vice' which – to use his own words – would 'rid England of this plague'. Nor was it just England: newspapers on this side of the Atlantic carried lengthy articles about a so-called 'Lavender Menace' in the United States.

Because the psychiatric community then regarded homosexuality as a mental illness, gay men and lesbians were considered susceptible to blackmail, thus constituting a security risk. Since this emerged at the same time as the notorious McCarthy witch-hunt against supposed communists, American government officials assumed that Soviet spies might blackmail homosexual employees of the federal government, who would provide them classified information rather than risk exposure.

At the same time as the US State Department 'allowed' 91 homosexuals to resign, the loathsome Senator McCarthy hired Roy Cohn – ironically, widely believed to be a closeted homosexual – as chief counsel of his Congressional subcommittee. Together, McCarthy and Cohn were responsible for the firing of scores of gay men from government employment, and strong-armed many opponents into silence using rumours of their homosexuality. This persecution of otherwise innocent gay men harmed many more people than the witch-hunt against communists. And it contributed greatly to the growing determination to persecute homosexuals in Britain.

To men like the Home Secretary, Lord Montagu

symbolised all that was good and bad in post-war British society: on the one hand he was of high aristocratic standing – educated at Eton, then Oxford, followed by service in the Grenadier Guards with a life even more privileged than most Peers. At the age of two, he had inherited Beaulieu, his family's 7,000-acre English estate, and a beautiful stately home known as Palace House. What's more he had almost single-handedly brought the upper class into the second half of the 20th century by challenging all aristocratic conventions and opening his home as a public tourist attraction in 1952. The public had proved to be fascinated and were extremely happy to pay to see what lay behind their secret walls. Very quickly, Beaulieu began generating revenue and Montagu's image shone as never before.

But on the other hand, the police and the Home Secretary knew that Edward Montagu was a self-confessed bohemian who enjoyed affairs with both men and women. To their minds, this undermined the very fabric of society: Baron Montagu was to be made an example of.

However, at his trial in December 1953 the jury was suspicious of what appeared to be clear indications that the police had tampered with the evidence. It dismissed one charge outright and left a second unresolved.

It is safe to say that the Home Secretary was not pleased. And so, before a projected retrial on the unresolved charge could occur, Lord Montagu was arrested once again: and this time the police meant to have their man once and for all.

At 7am on Saturday, 9 January 1954, Lord Montagu was in bed when the police came to arrest him. The Press had been tipped off and were already camped outside his house.

The Peer, his cousin Michael Pitt-Rivers and Peter Wildeblood, a prominent journalist, were charged with 'conspiracy to incite certain male persons to commit serious offences with male persons'.

It was the first time this charge had been used since the trial and imprisonment of Oscar Wilde in 1895: its use left me in no doubt that the police were pursuing a McCarthy-esque purge of society homosexuals.

Edward Montagu was, in fact, bisexual. While working for a London public relations firm he had met and enjoyed the company of Peter Wildeblood. But it was a friendship fraught with danger. Montagu was engaged to the American actress Anne Gage while Wildeblood was quite definitely gay. In the summer of 1953, Lord Montagu had offered Wildeblood the use of a beach hut near his country estate: Wildeblood brought with him two young RAF servicemen, Edward McNally and John Reynolds. The foursome were joined by Montagu's cousin Michael Pitt-Rivers.

What happened next was splashed all over the front pages of every newspaper in the country. At the trial the airmen, who had been exempted from all charges in exchange for their testimony, gave testimony about dancing and 'abandoned behaviour'. Montagu maintained that it was all remarkably innocent, although he later said that the men had enjoyed drinks, dancing and that 'we kissed'. But the director of public prosecutions appeared determined to secure a high-profile conviction and Aircraftsman McNally provided the prosecution with incriminating love letters written to him by Wildeblood. These were read out in court, full of the embarrassing endearments and sentimental language of a couple in love.

So severe was the law then that even something as tender as a love letter was enough to convict the defendants of the terrible crime of homosexuality. The three accused were sentenced to prison: Pitt-Rivers and Wildeblood, for 18 months each, while Montagu was sent down for 12 months.

As a high-profile member of the House of Lords, his conviction attracted huge media attention in virulently anti-homosexual Britain, and Edward's once-pristine reputation and promising career were all but ruined. The publicity surrounding the case also cost him his engagement.

Of the three, Lord Montagu was the only one to protest his innocence. He did so because he knew that he was innocent and that his conviction had been secured via guilt by association. The main evidence against the men was the love letters they had written. I heard a comment at the time that there was a slight smoke haze over London caused by all the gay men's love letters being burned.

This was a lesson homosexual men like me were only beginning to understand. For some years the police had routinely seized the diaries and telephone journals of men arrested for homosexuality. These were combed and used as the basis for more arrests: just being in the address book of a gay man was enough to tar you with the same brush. The Montagu case brought this home to us: if the police could fit up a Peer of the Realm in this way, what hope was there for the rest of us?

I, of course, had an additional reason to fear this Stalin-esque treatment. My name and Edward Montagu's were very similar and there was every chance, given the hostile climate of the time, that the police would jump to the (entirely wrong) conclusion that we were in some way linked. If so, then it wouldn't take much for them to discover my own secret life in the hazardous demi-monde of London homosexuality. It was a very frightening reminder of just how vulnerable I – and all those like me – were. Decades later I would have the chance to discuss this with my namesake in person – but in the summer of 1954 that was still a long way off, and my prevailing emotional was fear.

And yet in the appalling treatment meted out to Montagu, Pitt-Rivers and Wildeblood there was, unexpectedly, also hope. At the conclusion of the trial, and anticipating a hostile crowd outside the court, the police had kept the three men in the cells for two hours after the verdict. But when all three eventually emerged, to their surprise (and mine), they were greeted by cheers. Far from baying for their blood, the crowd clearly viewed them as martyrs.

And, evidently disturbed by the heavy sentences given to these highly respected public figures, *The Sunday Times* and some other leading newspapers published editorials questioning the wisdom of imposing such penalties for homosexual acts. For the first time gay men like me sensed the possibility of coming out of the closet: the trial of Lord Montagu and his associates had inadvertently nudged forward the movement for reform of the anti-gay laws. But it would be a long time coming.

The trial and imprisonment of my namesake for crimes of which I too was guilty was, of course, the appalling event of 1954. But something wonderful happened to me that year – something that went some way to drowning out the fear which affected all of us gay men. I fell in love.

I met Rodney through my first gay friend Steven. Rodney was only just 18 at the time. He was bright and very intelligent, having been to grammar school, but he was also very wise in the ways of the homosexual world: it was quickly clear that what he did not know about gays and the gay life wasn't worth knowing.

Rodney was naturally homosexual and told me he had known that this was the way he was built was since being a small boy. He was not obviously gay in any way, but all his family and friends knew and accepted the fact; I envied him that.

Rodney used to babysit for Steven's sister, so I saw him from time to time and always enjoyed talking to him, and gradually we started going out together. Some time later he told me that he had fallen in love with me almost the first day that he saw me: the date was 7.7.52 – seven was always my lucky number. I was 30 years old.

We would go up to London on a Saturday evening in my car, where he would show me gay clubs that I did not know about. Then he would sit in the car while I went in. Not only was he under 21 (the minimum admission age) but he also looked it.

During the summer we would drive to Brighton for the day on a Sunday, or sometimes for the weekend, Brighton being one of the most gay places outside London. There were several gay pubs and clubs in the town, and on the beach just where Brighton ends and Hove begins there was, in those days (and had been for many years apparently) a men-only part just between two breakwaters.

At the time Brighton was most widely known for being a place where heterosexual men would go with a girlfriend or a mistress. In the days of the old divorce laws where adultery had to be proved, it was the venue of choice for the evidence to be staged: there was a sort of semi-professional class of women co-respondents who, for a fee, would book into a B&B with the man seeking the divorce and arrange for a photographer to come and snap them in bed together. As a result no one really noticed the men-only area of the beach and on a good day it would get very full.

Strange as it may seem, in those days the authorities were totally unaware of this. There was not a great deal of homophobia in Brighton – largely, I think, because people just did not know very much about us, or indeed how many of us there were. And of course there was no gay press; nor was there was never anything written about us in the media except reports of arrests and convictions. With the exception of the Montagu trial these reports were always very brief and never made big headlines.

Most people did not yet have televisions and if even they did, homosexuality was never mentioned on the box, or on the radio. It would be more than a decade before the first hints of our existence troubled the placid waters of the BBC; and even when Jules and Sandy, two screamingly obvious gay characters, made their debut on the hit comedy show *Round The Horne* the subversive nature of their conversations were hidden in the old gay theatrical slang, or argot, of *Polari*.

No, in the 1950s we were underground – a subculture that was as yet largely undiscovered by the general public. And so, on that stretch of Brighton beach we would hold hands and cuddle (but no more than that): it was simply wonderful.

In the town were guesthouses owned by gays: all the rooms had double beds, and, of course, no questions were ever asked. I always looked forward to going to Brighton. But even so, we were careful to use a code: when I rang up to book, I would ask: 'Have you got a work bench vacant for the weekend?' It paid, as the Montagu trial had demonstrated all too vividly, to be careful.

During one of our weekend jaunts Rodney developed a problem with his big toe. He had to go into hospital where the doctors had to break and reset it. It surprised me to discover that he would have to convalesce there for more than a month. I visited him regularly and would find him sitting on the bed or chair with a spike down through the middle of his toe and a cork on the end of it. He was very bored.

One day I saw someone doing tapestry: they were happy to show me how easy it was and also told me it was a very therapeutic and time-passing hobby. Just the very thing for Rodney, I thought. And so I bought four small sample pieces, each about six inches square. Rodney took to it straight away and finished them all before he was discharged.

Sometime later I thought I must find a use for Rodney's tapestries. I had an idea. I made two more the same size featuring my crest, which I had carved onto the backs of my dining room chairs. I had 12 pieces of glass made, six of them an eighth of an inch larger all round, then had them laminated together. The next step was to make six frames in oak, mount the six tapestries and there I had six very permanent tablemats, where the glass was level with the top of the frames. That was more than 50 years ago and they have been used almost every day since.

Rodney being in hospital for that length of time was a problem for me and, I'm not proud to say that I was unfaithful. My sins (if that what they were) caught up with me: I picked up a sexually transmitted disease.

Gonorrhoea was very common in those pre-Aids days – amongst both straight and gay people. Most people unfortunate enough to catch it went surreptitiously to a special clinic, where they received (very anonymously) an injection of penicillin and all was well.

But once infected with gonorrhoea, it takes about six to nine days before you find out about it. In men this takes the form of a small yellow discharge from the penis. On one of my visits to see Rodney we had a kiss and a cuddle in the linen cupboard. He also gave me oral sex. That evening I was horrified to find that I was displaying signs of venereal disease – or VD. My first thought was: Bloody hell! Rod will have it in his stomach!

After rushing for advice to my friend Steven I was told to go and see a Dr Osmond Frank in Maidenhead. My friend telephoned him and explained the situation; he was told to tell me to go to his clinic and to wait until after the last patient had been seen. I saw the Doctor several times while I was waiting, he saw me and smiled reassuringly; I think he must have seen that I was very nervous. He was about 50, still quite handsome with red hair.

At last my turn came I went in and sat down in front of his desk. I told him of my problem and my fears, and he laughed. Then he told me something that I should have known if I had stopped to think about it, having done some basic study on anatomy and physiology. The acid juices in the mouth are very potent and kill most germs: there was no chance that I had infected Rodney.

As the doctor and I chatted, he asked me all about myself

in such a way that I suddenly realised that he, too, was gay. Then he got up and said: 'Follow me' and took me to the other side of the room where there were medical instruments. He said: 'Drop your trousers and let's have a look'. He gave me an injection of penicillin; and then he then became affectionate, dropped his own trousers and we had sex.

Soon after Rodney was discharged from hospital, he was called up to do his National Service. Although World War Two was fading into memory, Britain's army was involved in a number of overseas military operations – and was very short of numbers. And so the government introduced a law drafting all able-bodied men between the ages of 18 and 30 into the forces. They initially served for 18 months but in 1950, during the Korean War, this was increased to two years. The only official exemptions were blind and mentally ill people, clergymen and men in government positions abroad.

As a result I saw very little of Rodney for some time. Meanwhile Doctor Frank had taken something of a shine to me. He invited me to dinner at his house and I was very flattered to be asked: he was a very wealthy, well-educated man and I was even more impressed when he picked me up as arranged in a Rolls-Royce.

I expected to be taken to the large house, part of which was his surgery, but no, we drove to about halfway between Maidenhead and Bray, then into the driveway of an old beautiful large house on the banks of the Thames with a well-kept garden where the lawn swept down to the river. He showed me all over the house, which was full of antiques and oil paintings. We had drinks in the drawing room, which to my astonishment were served by a butler.

Dinner was a formal affair. The dining-room table was

about 12 feet long in heavy oak: it was laid for two, one at each end with real silver cutlery and candelabra. We talked a great deal and when I told Dr Frank about my singing, he said: 'I should love to hear you sing and with your permission, I should like to accompany you.' I had seen the grand piano in the drawing room and it turned out that my host was an accomplished pianist.

It was very plain to me that he was a very rich man and no ordinary doctor. I made enquiries and found that he was very well known, almost famous. He was the only man in the considerable history of Maidenhead who had been Mayor of the town for four years running, 1946 to 1950.

He was also married and had grown-up children; his wife was a senior psychiatric consultant at Windsor Hospital. And yet he made it clear that he had fallen in love with me. I must admit, I allowed myself to be seduced by this man: he took me around to places I could never have gone to and have never been to since, to the Ritz and the Junior Carlton Club, of which he was a member. He also took me to several art galleries. He taught me to improve my speech, my table manners, which piece of cutlery to use and when, the correct way to use a soup spoon. On one occasion I was asked to sing the solos at a choral concert with a large choir and orchestra. I needed a dinner jacket: Dr Frank bought it for me at Simpsons of Piccadilly, London.

I had designed my own crest that I intended to carve onto the backs of my dining-room chairs. Dr Frank said he wanted to buy me a ring and got me to have the size taken at a jeweller's. Then a few days later he presented me with a gold signet ring containing a large bloodstone onto which my crest was engraved, so that it could be used as a seal.

My relationship with Osmond Frank lasted about six months. He regularly took me to Brighton where we stayed at the upmarket Metropole Hotel. On one occasion we had planed to go to Brighton again to meet some friends, when at the last minute he was unable to go. Dr Frank told me to go on alone and take the 'Rolls'. I was astonished – and very thrilled. He had fallen very much in love with me. But the sad truth was that although I was very fond of him I did not love him: I was in love with Rodney.

Looking back, I think I must accept that with Dr Frank I was behaving a bit like a rent boy. Even at the time I felt very guilty, letting myself be spoilt by him – though it was not money but culture I craved from him. I still feel guilty about that period. It is difficult for me to face the truth and write about it, but I have promised myself that I will put it all down – the good and the bad – and let you, my readers, be my judge.

Throughout this time the police were very active in hunting down gays. They made regular and effective use of a local 'cottage' in my area. Officers hid in the loft area making a small hole at just the right spot to spy on those down below. Then they would arrest anyone they recognised as gay, even if they were not doing anything other than just standing there and not peeing. They would be charged with soliciting and convicted of gross indecency. And of course this would be fully reported in the local press and sometimes the national press too, so that the man's family would be devastated, often destroying a marriage and costing him his job.

There were several cases each week in just the Slough area alone; sometimes we heard that the man had committed suicide. But if this was reported in the press, there was often no mention of the original court case, despite this having been the reason for him taking his own life.

Still, I don't know how I would have got out of this relationship, had something tragic not happened. The local chief inspector of police for Maidenhead must have been informed that Dr Osmond Frank was gay. How he found out is sad in itself: there were at the time gay men who were also police informers. It was, as I say a very dangerous time for homosexuals.

This inspector was determined to arrest Dr Frank. And he decided the way to do so was to use his profession against him. A patient of his had gone to him with a complaint that required that Dr Frank, wearing a surgical glove to insect a finger into the boy's rectum. He was charged with sexual assault on the boy, who was then 17. I knew Osmond well by this time and that there was no possibility that he was a paedophile: but the police were out to get him.

It was a long and traumatic time before the case came to court. I was glad I had not broken off our relationship, something I had seriously thought about doing. We had to be very careful where we met now, but we did and I was glad to be able to give him some comfort and solace during his torment.

The prosecution's case was that what Dr Frank did was not medically required, and was therefore an indecent assault. Sir Peter Rawlinson, the top QC in the country at the time, was the defence barrister. The case lasted several days and it was plastered all over the national papers.

The jury, after an agonising time, failed to agree. The case was set down for a retrial, and all the evidence was given again. But the result was exactly the same: the jury members were split. Then, and only then, did the prosecution abandon the case.

Poor Osmond was a broken man – both in spirit and financially. He had aged 10 years and the case cost so much to defend that he had to sell his beautiful Thames-side house. He moved into the house where his surgery was and carried on for a while, but he lost most of his patients.

I felt so sorry for him. I telephoned him but he did not seem to want to see me. He was, as it turned out, being careful in case the beady and prejudiced eye of the police fell on me. I tried again several times, but got the clear impression he had told his secretary to tell me he was not in.

I was hurt but I understood. My hatred of the police at that time burned like a fire inside me. I had no truck with men who abused boys, but Dr Frank Osmond wasn't one of them. He had been crucified simply because he was homosexual.

EIGHT

The only good thing to come out of the whole sorry episode of Dr Frank's humiliation was the rekindling of my romance with Rodney.

When Rod was halfway though his national service he was transferred from Catterick in the north of England to Woolwich in London, which meant that we were able to see each other more often. Then, to his delight, he found that he could now live out from the barracks. We decided that this was the spur we needed: we would live together.

I suppose that as I write this today, in the enlightened climate of the 21st century, this may not seem such a big deal. But in 1955 it most certainly was. Official homophobia – and the arrests, convictions and imprisonments that exemplified it – was running hot. Two men setting up home together was not just them going against the law but wildly, daringly, thumbing their noses at it.

We looked around and found a cheap furnished room in Coleherne Road, Earls Court – then, as now, an area of London frequented by gays and with a reputation for being non-judgemental. We bought bits and pieces and made the little studio into the first home of our own that either of us had ever had.

I was, of course, still working ridiculously hard at my business, miles away in Berkshire. Nonetheless, we were determined that this would not stop us. And so every evening I would drive to Slough Railway Station and leave my car parked in the road right outside. Happily, there were no yellow lines or parking signs in those days. Catching a fast train to Paddington, then the Underground, I would be home in just an hour. And we were both deliciously happy together. We would get up at six in the morning and head off to our respective jobs – Rod to the army, me to my patternmaking.

On Sunday morning, if Rod was not on duty, we would have a lie-in – first time in my life I had lain in bed until nearly lunchtime. Then we would go for a drink to the pub at the end of the road. It was a typical London boozer called The Coleherne, and although it was a 'straight' pub during the week, we discovered that on Sunday mornings only there were quite a number of guys there in pairs just like us, as well as singles who would be 'cruising' (as looking for a sexual partner was, and still is, known). As a result we felt thoroughly at home.

During the year that we lived in the area we told all our friends about The Coleherne and on a Sunday morning the clientele became almost totally gay. More than 50 years later it has become a totally gay pub.

Long before my birth my great grandfather, Joseph

Montague, made a tapestry of Windsor Castle. It had been given to me during my childhood and I had noticed that woven into it was his name and the date – 1855. Since Rod had taken to tapestry so well, we decided we would like to do some together, to make something special for our home. We found a canvas with the conventional view of the castle painted on it, and for the rest of the year that we spent living in our little nest we worked to complete it. At the finish I wove both our names into the corner of the canvas, together with the date – 1955.

Our life together was wonderful. We were two people in love, contriving – in the face of hostile society and the law – to share a life. But sometimes the outside world, riddled as it was with prejudice, intruded. One evening Rod, who already hated every minute of his National Service, was very down. I asked: 'What's the matter, luv?' and he told me was he was suffering in the barracks. Apparently some of the other squaddies suspected that he was gay and were giving him a hard time, taunting him by saying, 'Come on Rod, let's have your bum.'

It could have been very dangerous. If the civilian world persecuted homosexuals, the army was even worse. But, danger or no danger, I wasn't having my lover tormented and I told him to stand up to them. 'Call their bluff, Rod – drop your trousers and say, "Come on then!"' It must have worked for Rod never again reported being bullied.

Then the day came when he was discharged. It was a day of mixed blessings because although it meant that he would be getting out of the army, the pressure was on for him to go back to live with his parents: we would lose our little home.

We were determined to stay living together. That year in

London, up to then, had been the happiest of both our lives. But how could we make it happen?

One of our gay friends was the owner of a very large chain of building societies. We approached him, told him of our dilemma and to our delight he offered us a beautiful flat in Beaconsfield, South Buckinghamshire. It was a detached building with a large car park at the front, a road on either side, a large spare piece of ground at the back and two shops underneath. It was a unique shape: it had five equal sides, so we called it The Pentagon.

Rodney began working for Slough Town Council, but he didn't settle in well and the pay was very poor. So I managed to get him a job working for a customer of mine as the accountant. These were the days of pounds, shillings and pence and no calculators, but Rodney was a natural: he could add up a long row of figures quicker than anyone I ever knew. The manager, who was an alcoholic, relied on Rod totally. Before long he was running the office and managing the works all on his own – with a little discreet help behind the scenes from me.

Sexually, our life was very special. We were not conventional (even if a homosexual relationship could then have been described as conventional). We had an open relationship, meaning that we could (and did) see other people. But there were no secrets and although I was never completely faithful to Rod he said he was never jealous. Years later, however, I found that he could remember the names of every one of my 'one night stands' as we called them (although I rarely slept all night with any of them).

Before long our life became even less conventional – and considerably more dangerous: John came to live with us.

John was 17 when we first met him through one of our discreet circle of gay friends. He had discovered he was gay at the age of 15 and had had a relationship with someone we knew. He was an only child and did not get on too well with his father who was old enough to be his grandfather. When John's lover dumped him, he began visiting us for consolation and company.

I was very concerned at this development, but felt I could not turn him away: I suppose I became a bit of a father figure to this lonely young man. I remember telling him that he was too young to decide he was homosexual and that – as many others have found – he might be going through a phase. I also was very aware that the situation was dangerous. It was 1957, and not only was any homosexuality still against the law, but the fact that he was so young could raise very uncomfortable questions.

John spent a great deal of time with us, often spending the night and the weekend. As we had only one bedroom and one bed he slept on the couch, but eventually took to creeping into bed with us. A little after his 18th birthday he moved in with us. We were now a threesome and, perhaps inevitably, we had sex – though only in our flat; because of his age we never took John to any gay venue.

Oddly, one day someone gave John a nickname – Tuptim. It's an unusual word, the name of the second wife of the king of Siam, but it somehow stuck. In one of the strange coincidences that have happened throughout my life, many years later I was to meet and entertain in my London flat a Thai Princess who turned out to be a direct descendant of the real Princess Tuptim.

During this time I was producing the Burnham District Scout Gang Show. John had been a Scout and now he was an adult he signed up as an Assistant Scout Leader. He helped me at the hospital with my group and enjoyed taking part in the Gang Shows. One particular sketch we did was the 'Floral Dance'. I sang and John dressed up as a girl, as did most of the straight men in the show at some time. John looked every inch a pretty girl and we danced the Floral Dance together on stage in front of a packed audience including many of our gay friends.

That year, 1957, was a seismic one for homosexuals in Britain. Prompted, in part, by the public condemnation of the trial of Lord Montagu, a committee of the great and good had been examining the laws on homosexuality for three years. Led by the former headmaster of Uppingham and Shrewsbury public schools, Sir John Wolfenden, a panel of 12 men and three women had interviewed gay men about their lives and their treatment by the law. It was a sign of the times that the committee's remit was to enquire into homosexuality and prostitution – the two seemingly inextricably linked in the establishment mind – and that to spare the women members' blushes it adopted peculiarly English code words: homosexuals were to be referred to as 'Huntleys' and prostitutes as 'Palmers'. Only in Britain could something so serious be disguised with the name of a famous brand of biscuits.

Getting gay men to give evidence was of considerable difficulty for the committee. Wolfenden considered placing an advert in a newspaper or magazine, but the committee instead decided to locate three men willing to give evidence. One of them was Peter Wildeblood who had been imprisoned with Lord Montagu in the infamous 1954 trial. The three witnesses were also given pseudonyms to protect their identities.

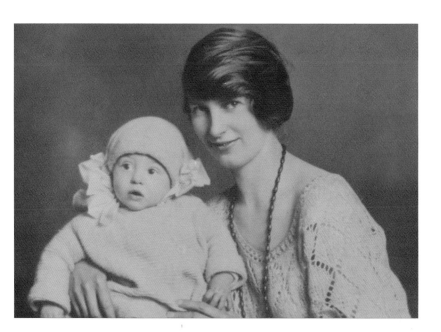

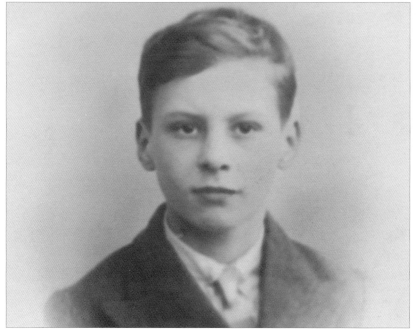

Above: Me with my mother, Nellie, in 1923.

Below: Me aged about 8 in my Taplow village school uniform.

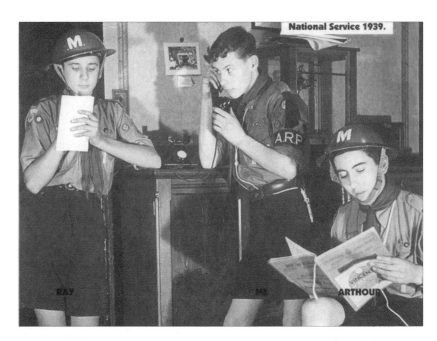

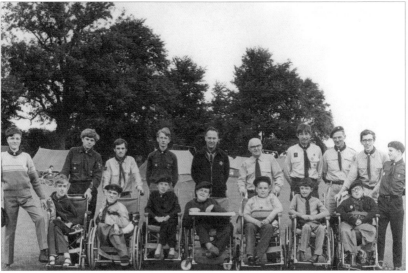

Above: I was proud to be a Boy Scout and here I am providing a telephone answering service for the Home Guard during my national service.

Below: I was part of the Scout movement for many years and set up the first Scout unit for profoundly disabled boys, enabling them to enjoy many aspects of Scouting, including camps. I ran this unit for 25 years.

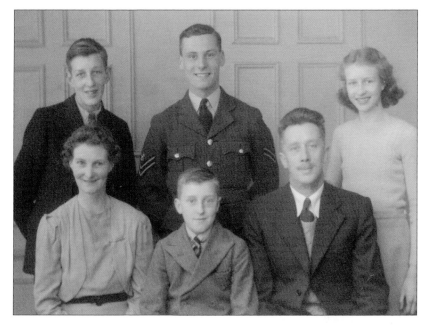

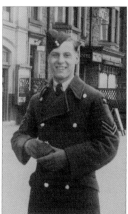
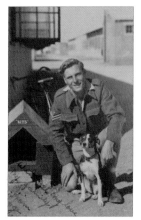
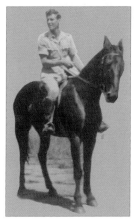

Top: I enlisted into the RAF in May 1941. Here I am top middle with my brother Edward on my right and sister Elizabeth on my left. My mother, Nellie, brother John and father George are in front.

Below left: In Blackpool in 1942.

Below centre: I served in Rhodesia for three years. Here I am with my pet dog, Bits.

Below right: Always a keen horseman I had my own horse, Oscar, while serving in Rhodesia.

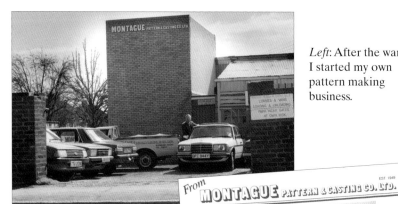

Left: After the war I started my own pattern making business.

Right: We celebrated its 40th anniversary in 1989.

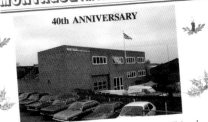

Left: I became a choir boy at age 7 and continued all my life. Here I am in the Burnham Village Choir in 1948.

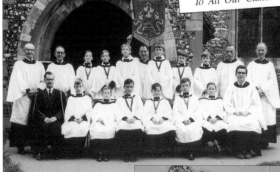

Right: I was very moved when my singing teacher, Harold Mead presented me with this wonderful watercolour of me singing.

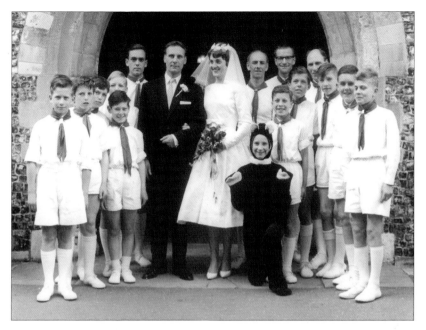

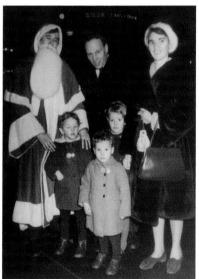

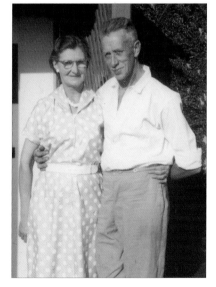

Above: On the 27th May 1961 I married Vera in Burnham church.

Below left: I loved family life: here we are visiting Father Christmas in Selfridges in 1967. My children Martin, Edward and Paula are L-R in front of me.

Below right: My mother, Nellie and father, George, outside their house in 1967.

Right: I love new challenges and as the children began to grow up I decided to build my own boat. Woody soon became an important part of our family.

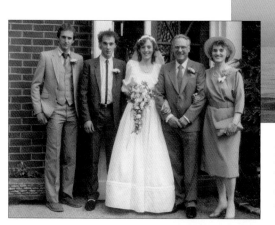

Left: In 1985 my daughter Paula got married. Here we all are on the day. L-R Martin, Edward, Paula, me and Vera.

Right: Me with my grandchildren. L-R Daniel, Kimberley and Simon.

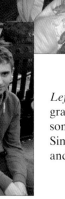

Left: With my grandchildren again some years later. L-R Simon, Kimberley and Daniel.

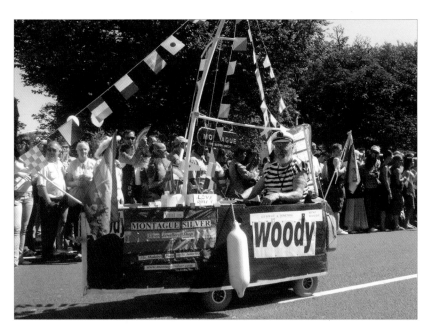

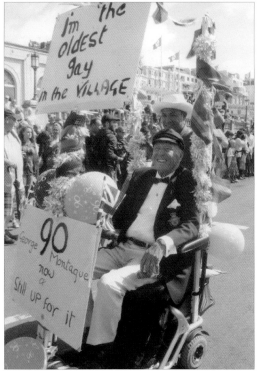

Above: I had come out to my family in 1982 but it was some years before I took part in my first Gay Pride march. Here I am in 2007.

Left: By 2013 they had made me ambassador!

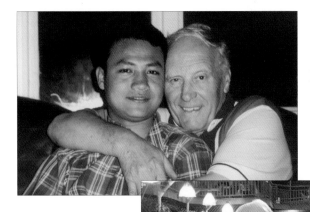

Left: I met Somchai, the love of my life, in 1997.

Right: With Somchai in Thailand in 2012.

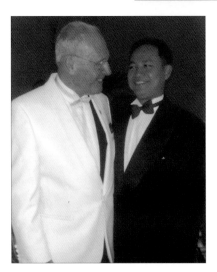

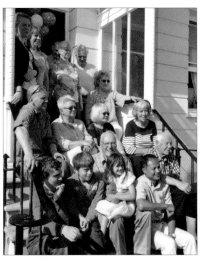

Bottom left: On 15th April 2006 we celebrated our relationship by entering a civil partnership.

Bottom right: Surrounded by friends and family on the steps to our flat celebrating my 90th birthday in June 2013. It was a very special occasion.

Wolfenden's report was published on 4 September 1957 – and it caused a sensation. Disregarding the conventional ideas of the day, the committee found that 'homosexuality cannot legitimately be regarded as a disease, because in many cases it is the only symptom and is compatible with full mental health in other respects.'

With all but one member in agreement, the committee recommended that 'homosexual behaviour between consenting adults in private should no longer be a criminal offence'. And its report added this ringing proclamation of the right of consenting adults to find love with whoever they chose.

'The law's function is to preserve public order and decency, to protect the citizen from what is offensive or injurious, and to provide sufficient safeguards against exploitation and corruption of others...

'It is not, in our view, the function of the law to intervene in the private life of citizens, or to seek to enforce any particular pattern of behaviour.'

On the surface this looked like a red-letter day for homosexuals. However, the committee made clear that it regarded homosexuality as a debilitating condition, which should be treated, if possible, by medical means. It also strongly opposed decriminalisation of public homosexual acts, and recommended stiff penalties for male prostitution. For good measure it suggested that the age of consent for homosexual acts should be 21, rather than 16, as it was for heterosexual (or even lesbian) sex.

Wolfenden's conclusions apparently came as a shock to the government (an indication, perhaps, that it had not really done its homework before appointing him: his son was widely known to be gay). Clouds of homophobia trailed in its wake with leading politicians and judges contesting the philosophical basis and practical outcomes of the proposed decriminalisation of homosexuality. It was, therefore, less than surprising that the government delayed and dithered over whether to enact Wolfenden's key recommendations. In fact, the only concrete outcome of the whole report was a new law, in 1959, to make male prostitution and street solicitation (by both men and women) illegal. It was a clear case of one step forward, two steps back.

To campaign for the Wolfenden proposals, a small group of both straight and gay supporters of reform discreetly founded the Homosexual Law Reform Society. By 1959, the HLRS had begun to launch a nationwide campaign to end the legal persecution of gay men.

And what was I doing while all this was going on? Perversely, I was thinking of going straight.

Rod and I had been together for five years. Perhaps inevitably, we had started to grow apart and go our own ways. John now had a girlfriend and the more we thought about it, the more he and I realised we wanted to get married (though not, of course, to each other) – we wanted conventional family lives. But Rod was 100 per cent gay and was in the process of getting on the housing ladder by buying his own house in Slough. Our time together was drawing to a close.

I was now 36 and for some time I had been putting up with a great deal of subtle pressure to get married. Mum, in particular, kept dropping little hints. She was very wise and I'm sure she had an idea of the kind of life I was leading.

During the very sad moments of Dr Frank's trial we talked abut him and she knew he had been an influence in my life. On one occasion I was upset and started to talk to her about it. She must have guessed that I was going to tell her that I was gay, for she said: 'If one of my sons were like that, I would rather that he did not tell me.'

(Since then I have always advised people that have asked me whether to tell their mother of their sexuality that they should not do so – unless she specifically asks. My reasoning for this is that if you tell her, you put her on the spot: she has to say something in response and may not be ready to. In any event, mothers are usually very wise where their offspring are concerned. She probably knows anyway.)

I had met Vera through my business. She was working for a customer of mine and for several years I had seen her almost every day. Somehow it seemed natural for us to become a couple. I was honest with her from the start; I explained my homosexual past and the fact that I had lived with Rodney for several years. She accepted it and, as time wore on, we grew to love each other.

We had a very short engagement. As soon as my family and friends got to hear that we were fiancés, they started to organise the wedding. I would not be telling the truth if I didn't admit that I thoroughly enjoyed the events leading up to the big day, as well as the marriage ceremony itself. And it was wonderful to see Mum so happy. She and Dad were truly in their element. Since Vera and I were now in our 30s – and because of my business and Scouting life – we knew so many people that the invitation list was never-ending.

The one set of friends I did not involve were those from my old life. From the time I got engaged I cut myself off completely from all my gay friends. Rodney was the sole exception. He supported me totally, as he always did with everything – his love for me was so complete that all he wanted was my happiness – but he told me that most of our old crowd did not approve of what I was doing.

I had been in the Burnham Village Choir for some time, so the whole choir turned up, and with them the bell ringers. Without my knowledge a large group of my singing friends got together to rehearse a piece to sing at the service. It was beautiful. And when we came out of the church there was a guard of honour with lads from the Gang Show dressed in the Scouts Gang uniform.

The reception was held in a large marquee at my parents' house. In all, 150 guests attended and I was kept so busy that I learned to shake hands with two people at once. It's probably something I first learned in the Scouts, where you shake hands with the left hand.

For the honeymoon we toured Spain in my Alpha Romeo sports car, going through places where very few tourists venture: wherever we stopped, the locals just stood in groups and looked at us. On arriving home we settled into my small one-bedroomed flat in Beaconsfield.

Are you wondering, at this stage, how such a transformation was possible? How did a man who had discovered his homosexuality – and not just discovered it but embraced and celebrated it – suddenly become a heterosexual husband? To put it bluntly, did the mechanics of marriage work?

The answer to the first question is that I made conscious decision to be a full-time husband. For over four years from the day I got married I led a totally heterosexual lifestyle. I very much enjoyed it and was proud to introduce people to 'my wife'. I enjoyed the sound of the words and loved the feeling of being in our relationship. I also made a promise to Vera that whatever happened I would never leave her until the children were adults.

And the answer to the second? In just a year our daughter Paula was born. I turned a very small boxroom into a nursery. It was so small that it was not much bigger than the cot. Then within another few months our first son, Martin, was on the way.

Paula had been born in hospital, but Martin was born at my parents' house. I revelled in fatherhood. Martin was a very long time emerging, so I took Vera outside, walking her round and round. And it seemed to work; eventually Martin arrived in the world. I'm proud to say that I was present at the birth of both Martin and Paula.

And I loved the responsibility of having a family. Our little flat was on the first floor with a large area of flat roof at the same level. It was also not terribly convenient: the pram had to be kept in a shed at the bottom of the steps. This was a problem for Vera as it involved carrying Paula up the steps and then returning to carry the baby up, then once again for the shopping, all up and down the same steps. Something had to be done.

At the back of the property was a piece of waste ground. so I built a 40-foot-long ramp with small steps in the middle. There were planks either side for the wheels of the pram. The gradient worked out at one in four, so enabling Paula and most of the shopping to go up in one trip, then, with a bit of an effort, Vera could just about manage to push the pram with baby Martin in it up the ramp.

It wasn't long before our third child was on the way. Now we knew would have to find a bigger house. We were lucky to find one only half a mile away from my works and with two schools nearby. Edward was born in our new home and I then spent all the time I could spare – after the Gang Shows and being with my troop of Scouts at the hospital – working on our new home.

We needed somewhere to store the coal for the central heating, as well as a small workshop, a garden toolshed, plus a playroom. I combined the lot in one attractive building with a pitched roof covered in cedar tiles. With the material left over I built a Wendy house. The next job was kitchen units, after that an extension to the kitchen for use as a laundry. I had become a fully-fledged husband and father.

I looked forward to seeing the children each evening, helping with bath times and bed times. I got a great feeling of belonging again, especially at family gatherings with the children of my brother and two sisters. And the total happiness of my mother was plain to see. We all gathered at my parents' house each Christmas. I was proud to sit next to my father in his place as the head of the family. I belonged – and it felt marvellous.

Was I a good father? As good as, or better than, a 'normal' heterosexual man? I like to think so. Every so often there is a debate about smacking children. All I can say is that we never found it necessary. Vera and I impressed on them that if they were good in public we would forgive them a great deal in the house. There was just the occasion when the boys were about a year old and sitting in their highchairs at the table. They started to throw the food on the floor, look at me in defiance – and then do it again.

I picked up a tablespoon and said. 'If you do that again I shall punish you and you will cry.' They duly did it again – and I duly (and carefully) gave a measured tap with the back of the spoon on their knuckles. They never did it again, and while they were very young, if they ever misbehaved at the table I would pick up the spoon. When I did so they would put their hands under the table, but we never had to repeat the treatment.

I took a lot of film with my 8mm cine camera, capturing all the family weddings, christenings, birthdays and holidays. But I got fed up with setting the screen up in the lounge every time to show them. I wanted a small cinema for us, as a family, to enjoy these moments. I also needed a study, so I combined the two.

The room I built was about 20 feet by 10. It replaced an old and much smaller shed (planning permission was not so strict in those days) and everything was in wood with a pitched roof. The windows came from my village church, left over from an extension there. I constructed a small projection room, complete with a small window just like a real cinema. Vera and the children were thrilled.

From the outside I would defy anyone to look at us and not believe we were a regular, conventional family. And I'm not ashamed to say that I loved creating things for our home. When I had come home from the war I had seen in the estate woodshed a large pile of oak 'in stick' – wide planks of wood with thin sticks between each one, so that it 'air dries' thoroughly. I had a plan for these, and one day I asked Dad about them.

He told me that during the war, one of the best oak trees in the park had been commandeered by the government to build the frames of Mosquito bomber aeroplanes. The state was not required to pay for this lumber, but once it had all been through the sawmill they returned a quarter of the wood to the estate, which apparently planned to use it for firewood.

Even in those days the value of this beautiful oak would be several hundred pounds. I went up to the Hall and asked the Colonel – Dad's employer – if he would sell it to me. He was plainly intrigued and asked what I planned to do with it. I told him that I wanted to build my own dining-room furniture – and was astonished by the response: 'Then you shall have it, my boy, with my compliments.'

Over the next year or so whenever I had a few spare hours outside the working day I would plug away on it. I first built a small coffee table and two stools as a model, followed by a large Cromwellian-style table with eight chairs – two armchair type and six in a milking stool style.

I designed the whole suite including two sideboards, and when finished I engraved my own crest on the backs of the chairs – a naked cubit arm symbolic of a manual worker (me!) and a sprig of Mountain Ash. I couldn't have know it then, but there would come a time when – in the pits of despair – this experience of working in wood and creating something solid and reliable would help restore my sanity.

And so, as the '60s – that decade of hedonism and self-expression – progressed I drowned myself in family life, work and my beloved Scouting. The only person from my past life with whom I kept in touch was Rodney. I would take the children around to his house, and he – knowing that he would never marry or have children of his own – enjoyed seeing mine grow up.

But although every waking hour was totally taken up with my work, the family and Scouting, I began to yearn for homosexual contact. Despite all the sublimation of my desires – and all three of the demands on my time were, I now see, unquestionably acts of sublimation – I could not control my thoughts or the feelings in my groin.

At the time I was doing a lot of travelling on business. Two or three times a week I would drive hundreds of miles in all directions. And as I sat in my car, pursuing my dream of a normal life, my sex drive was as high as ever.

At all the toilets that I had to pass along the route there was, without exception, temptation. There were no real motorways or service stations in those days, but there were toilets specifically built for travellers, miles from anywhere, generally situated in dual carriageway lay-bys. There were always at least half a dozen lorries, vans and cars parked up – and at least half of the drivers of these would be loitering either inside or outside looking for sex.

Most of these buildings were made of wood, including the cubicles, which always had holes two or three inches in diameter between them. These had been created by the men who visited them: brief and generally anonymous relief was to be found by pushing your penis through the aperture and into the welcoming hands or mouth of the person on the other side.

Was I alone in being tempted? Was it only inveterate homosexuals who patronised them? No, and no. I'm positive that most of the loiterers would be just like me: married men with a wife and children at home, men who would not consider themselves to be homosexual or bisexual and were more likely be homophobic at their works or in the pub.

For a long time I managed to resist the temptation that was there. It was, I confess, a struggle. A friend who was just like me, married but once gay, said despairingly of his desires: 'That bloody thing between my legs!' I knew exactly what he meant. I suffered mental and physical agonies in my fight with my unruly desires. I would go for hours without peeing rather than stopping at these places – and would eventually urinate in a lay-by where there was no toilet and no temptation. But eventually my resolve was not strong enough.

I began to give in, quickly entering the toilets, finding a cubicle, doing it quickly and walking out full of shame. For a short while after each visit I would hate myself. Then I would make my mind forget about it and pretend it had not happened. Until the next time. The only thing that always put me off was very normal, good looking guys who, when they took down their overalls had black silk stockings and suspenders on, and asked you if you had any pictures of naked women.

And so gradually, I once again began living a double life, with all the dangers and all the nervous strain that went with it. It couldn't continue: something was bound to give.

NINE

It was now midway through the 1960s. A new era had dawned, an age not just of rock and roll (which had arrived in Britain almost a decade before and almost without me noticing) but one in which the whole warp and weft of society was undergoing enormous change. The introduction of the contraceptive pill in 1961 had led, inexorably, to the loosening of traditionally restrictive attitudes to sex. And the Age of Aquarius – a time of experimentation, drugs, hippies and the wholesale rejection of the hidebound attitudes and prejudices of the post-war years – was upon us.

And how did George Montague, successful businessman (for my company had grown and was now employing a significant workforce at a new site), husband, father, Scout leader and conflicted homosexual, fit in to this new era? With difficulty, that's how.

I was devoting huge amounts of time to Scouting. By 1962 there were only about a dozen boys of Scout and Cub age left on the hospital unit. Rheumatic fever, like polio had been virtually eliminated. Those lads remaining had rheumatism-related problems, such as Still's disease and chorea.

In December that year I was appointed Assistant County Commissioner (Extension Activities) Buckinghamshire – the title recognised that I was now responsible for Scouting for boys with a handicap. I handed over to my senior assistant, who carried on for another six years, until the unit closed.

I estimated that during my time there, at least 500 boys either joined, or continued Scouting – an achievement of which I was very proud. On four occasions we had a representative in the corner of the quadrangle at the St Georges Day Parade, Windsor Castle. This is where all those boys who have passed the Queen's Scout Badge are inspected by, and then march past, a member of the Royal Family. Most often this was Her Majesty the Queen.

It was around then, on seeing a boy in a wheelchair in an able-bodied troop – completely at home and accepted by all – that a driving force stirred within me to do more for handicapped boys, particularly those in wheelchairs.

Nationally it was government policy for kids with a handicap, particularly those in wheelchairs, to be sent to special schools. I thought that in many cases this was simply wrong, and I could see no reason why many of those confined to a wheelchair should not attend an ordinary school, or participate in the weekly able-bodied Scout troop night.

Some years earlier we had begun a camp for our disabled lads at Dorneywood – a very grand 18th-century mansion and extensive grounds at Burnham. The house itself has long been assigned as the country seat of a senior member of the government – usually the Chancellor of The Exchequer. It is now owned and managed by the National Trust, having been given to the nation in 1947 by Lord Courtauld-Thomson.

During one weekend district camp, his Lordship had paid us a visit. I took the opportunity to buttonhole him and make a case for us to be allowed to continue to use the lovely site since Scouting was growing in the district. I also stressed how important camping was as part of the Scout training. He reassured me that, after his death, we would be taken care of and able to use the grounds as a permanent camp.

But when his lordship died I discovered that nothing had been done to ensure this. The National Trust agent told us that there were no instructions in the will regarding our use of the site, and as the house was going to be used by the Foreign Secretary he doubted we would be allowed to use it. Security concerns were cited as the main reason, but he also said he was worried about fire and damage to trees. I pointed out to him the importance of youth training. I told him that we taught boys about these things. He said we could continue for the time being.

It was a tenuous arrangement and I was concerned – the camp had become increasingly important, not just to me but to the lads for whom I was responsible. And before long something happened to make me more nervous still.

In the wood behind the campsite we discovered a large ring of rhododendrons and azaleas that in the early spring were, for several weeks, a blaze of colour. On talking to one of the gardeners from the Dorneywood house we were told that his Lordship had planted this area many years before as a place where he could go to sit and contemplate in perfect peace and quiet.

We asked if we could use this circle as our Scout Chapel, in return for keeping the area – which had become somewhat overgrown – in good order. His Lordship had no hesitation in giving us his blessing, saying that although he could no longer get up there he was pleased for us to use it, particularly for that purpose. We used some granite blocks given to us by the local council to erect an altar on which we placed a cross made out of silver birch. But this led to a wild and dangerous story in the press.

A little while after we had erected the altar I had a call from a friend who said: 'Have you seen what the local paper is saying about the chapel?' Apparently someone out trespassing – for this was a private wood – had seen our altar, told the local newspaper and a reporter had written an article suggesting it was connected with black magic. It even suggested that our Scout Chapel could be the site of a modern day 'hellfire club' – the notorious 18th-century organisation of society rakes (as the dissolute aristocracy was then known) to conduct pagan sex rites, orgies and satanic black masses. It was, of course, the most ridiculous nonsense and, fortunately, didn't lead anywhere. But it was also a sharp reminder to me of the way rumours, particularly when they involved sex, could be dangerous, especially when they involved the Scouts.

Eventually we got full permission for a permanent site at Dorneywood. Plans went in for toilets, a camp wardens' hut, a providore (Scout tuck shop) and also a permanent hut as a dormitory.

The whole area around the camp had, at the beginning of the century, been a brick works with its own kiln, the remains of which could still be seen. Three very large craters remained. The largest was about 60 feet across and 20 feet deep, presumably where the clay had been dug out. Over the course of three years, we converted this crater into one of the finest campfire circles in the country. I wore out my little company pick-up truck moving about 50 tons of granite from a local dump to be placed in tiers just like a Roman amphitheatre. When we had finished it could seat more than a thousand.

After three years hard work by everyone I could persuade or press-gang to help, the camp was ready for its opening day. In the meantime, someone put us in touch with HP Baked Beans. They wanted to make a commercial for television and needed 200 Cub Scouts. I contacted the producer and suggested that they do it at Dorneywood. He visited the site and was very impressed, deciding there and then to use the campfire circle.

I duly arranged it all with the local Cub packs, and on the day a film crew of at least 40 with mountains of equipment and a large catering van arrived. Then along came three large coaches and many cars packed with excited Wolf Cubs. The producer asked that they be assembled in the campfire circle so that he could tell them what he wanted them to do. If you have ever seen 200 lads of that age together you can imagine the noise. He tried to make himself heard so that he could start, but was getting no attention. So, with my drill instructor's voice I shouted: 'Pack, Pack, Pack'. (The first thing a Cub learns is to be quiet when a Cub Scout Leader shouts that.) Immediately there was complete silence; the producer was amazed.

After they had dished out 200 plates of baked beans they started filming, but before long it started to rain. I told them I did not think it would clear up that day. This turned out to be a blessing for us as it all had to be done again the following weekend. This meant that we got the fee I had negotiated, plus a further 50 per cent for the repeat performance and all expenses paid. We received £450, all of which was spent on improvements and getting the camp ready for the official opening in the summer of 1963. The only upset of the whole event was an outbreak of tummy upset amongst some of the Cubs, caused by eating too many beans. But after a few weeks they were all able to watch themselves on television, and the commercial was shown for about six weeks.

There is a reason for me telling you all this. I was devoting all my spare time – and quite a few of my working hours – to Dorneywood and the Scouts. In summer and winter I would be there weekend in, weekend out. Much of this time should, of course, have been spent concentrating on my business or with my family, but immersing myself in the Scouts was a way to sublimate my troublesome sexual desires, and the enormous efforts I made on behalf of the movement would only serve to sharpen the pain I would, in time, feel when it eventually betrayed me.

It was a former Chief Scout, the late Lord Somers, who wrote: 'To help a lame dog over the stile is considered to be one of the primary virtues, but to teach that lame dog to climb over the stile by himself – particularly if the lame dog happens to be a boy with a handicap – is even better.'

I was determined to do something to ease the plight of disabled lads who would benefit from the full experience of being a Scout. But how? I heard of the *London Agoonoree*, a camp run specifically for handicapped boys from London. I wrote and asked if I could join the 1964 camp. It would be the first of four camps that I was to attend – and each time I was able to take some of the disabled lads from my Scout Troop along.

But by the 1967 camp, held in Belgium, it was clear that the *Agoonoree* was getting too big and that it could no longer take boys from outside the London area. The organisers suggested that I start my own camp. It was a daunting prospect. I had gained a great deal of knowledge at these *Agoonoree* camps, but being in charge of a patrol of eight severely physically handicapped boys with eight other able-bodied boys of about the same age as 'buddies' (helpers), for eight days was, was another matter altogether.

It would need a dormitory, at least one State Registered Nurse, transport, a bus with a tail lift, a mountain of equipment, a central kitchen, trained staff – and, naturally, funds. To make a camp of this nature viable we would have to amalgamate with other counties. I wrote to five neighbouring counties and got favourable replies from all of them. I was overwhelmed at the thought of the organisation involved. But I had a strange feeling, a mixture of destiny and heavy responsibly, together with a realisation that this was something that simply had to be done, and at that moment I was the only one who would do it. And I knew, too, that if I did not follow it up, there would be no camp for disabled Scouts outside London.

Somehow we made it work. It is one of the things about which I am most proud – that for many years following our first camp, disabled lads enjoyed and benefited from the extraordinary camaraderie of the Scouting environment. The motto of our first camp was 'doing'. It was important that these lads, who had become used to just sitting and having everything done for them, should be doing for themselves not just watching, so we trained the helpers to be on constant watch, and wherever possible (and often even if it seemed impossible) our disabled Scouts had a go at everything an able-bodied boy would have done.

So immersed in the demands of this voluntary effort did I become that I'm not sure I noticed what was happening in the world outside. But much was happening nonetheless: the world, particularly for homosexual men, was about to change. And for once, it was changing for the better.

The brutal and discriminatory laws that turned our desires into criminal offences had not been changed one jot in the years since the Wolfenden Report. However, public opinion had shifted. The spur was probably the lifting, in 1958, of a ban on the treatment of homosexual topics in the theatre. Prior to then, the Lord Chamberlain's office could – and did – simply censor out of existence anything that had a gay theme.

By the early 1960s, a number of plays and films dealt openly with homosexual issues. One film was particularly important in promoting reform: *Victim*, released in 1961, starred Dirk Bogarde as a barrister whose career and marriage were threatened by a blackmailer aware of his homosexual activities. Then in 1964, the BBC, which had traditionally been hostile to anything gay, presented a sensitive full-length documentary comparing the lives of homosexual men in the UK with those in the Netherlands.

Despite these sympathetic films newspapers consistently characterised gay men as pathetic creatures, and emphasised the threat they posed because of the fear of blackmail. Nor was that fear entirely groundless: in the autumn of 1962, public attention was riveted by the highly publicised trial of William Vassall, a Foreign Office clerk, accused of providing classified information to a KGB agent who had taken compromising photographs of him. It was an extreme example of what all of us with dangerous sexual desires knew could ruin us at any moment.

And the police were still hunting us down in evermore extreme ways. In Hertfordshire, police removed floorboards from the main floor of Baldock Town Hall so that they could spy on the toilets below. Even an apparent attempt to rein them in by the Director of Public Prosecutions was, in reality, a cynical smokescreen. In 1964 he ordered that all chief constables obtain consent before bringing charges for sexual acts between men in private. Rather than an attempt to improve the lives of gay men, however, this change was really intended to counter the protests of gay campaigners about the uneven application of the law of the land. The arrests continued unabated.

But Labour's victory in the 1966 general election heralded real change, or at least the promise of it. The new government introduced a homosexual law reform bill. But to get it through the House of Commons would require a great deal of political manoeuvring. The government scheduled the debate on the bill to run without interruption from the afternoon of 3 July into the early hours of the next day. It was a tactic designed to wear down the will of opponents and by the time the final vote was taken, significant numbers of exhausted members had left the House. Finally, the Sexual Offences Bill finally was passed shortly after dawn on the morning of 4 July 1967 and, with the granting of Royal Assent on 28 July, the bill became law.

But what, in reality, did the new law do? Not as much as you might think – or anywhere near what we'd hoped for and needed.

Yes, it finally decriminalised sex between two consenting male adults. But the age at which – for the purposes of this law and this law only – a man became an adult was set at 21. This was not just five years older than that for heterosexual activity, but it was also three years older than the voting age, the age at which you could buy alcohol or cigarettes, and five years above the age at which a boy could join the army.

To make matters worse, the maximum penalty for any man over 21 committing acts of 'gross indecency' (which included masturbation and oral sex) with a 16- to 21-year-old was increased from two years to five years. And that offence of gross indecency – brought in by the hateful Labouchère Amendment back in Victorian times – still applied. This meant that same-sex relations were legal only in private (unlike, again, heterosexual activities), which was interpreted as being behind locked doors and windows – and with no other person present anywhere on the premises.

And while gay sex itself was now legal, most of the things that might lead to it were still classified as 'procuring' and 'soliciting'. What that meant in practice was that it remained a crime for two consenting adult men to chat up each other in any non-private location. Farcically – or, more accurately, tragically – it was even illegal for two men to exchange phone numbers in a public place or to attempt to contact each other with a view to having sex. Therefore, the 1967 law – supposed to be the great liberalising act of Parliament – established the bizarre anomaly that to arrange to do something now legal was itself illegal.

Why did this matter to me, aside from its manifest injustice? Because despite my best efforts to constrain my sexuality something dramatic had happened in my life. I had fallen in love, again.

I had been married for six years. My wife knew about my lifestyle and some of my gay friends before we got married. She knew I had lived with my boyfriend in the very flat where we lived after the wedding. But we hadn't discussed it as much as we should have done. Nobody did then; and many people still do not today.

We had both wanted to get married, and we had both wanted children. Vera had been 29 at the time of our wedding; I was 37. Looking back, I cannot regret what we did, for our children were a blessing and a delight. But we were young and, with so little reliable information about homosexuality in the public domain, believed that my past life could stay that way: an aberration to be brushed over, forgotten or ignored. After all I had been attracted to women before and I had assured my new bride – as I assured myself – that I was determined to give up the gay life style. But it came to dawn on me that although I loved Vera, I was not 'in love' with her.

Then I met Michael. The circumstances in which we came to meet were typically complex – and I say typical because, in those days gay encounters were often remarkably awkward and chance affairs.

I had sex with a man who told me that he was not gay, but happened to remark that his brother was. Some time later I had an occasion to visit him at his home, where he introduced me to his two brothers. David and Michael. I asked him which was the gay one and he told me it was David. Wrong. I later met Michael in circumstances where it was clear that he was the gay one; in fact, his first words were: 'You won't tell my brothers, will you...'

The law had now changed so it was no longer an offence for two men to have sex if it was in private and there was no other person present. Before long Michael became my lover.

Michael was a milkman, starting very early in the morning, and would finish work by lunchtime. I gave him a part-time job at my company driving the van and other jobs in the works. He worked very hard. I admired him; I fell in love with him. He told me all about his life and his family: his mother was mentally ill, and his father was dying of lung cancer.

He told me that he and his brothers had all been sexually abused from about the age of 11 or 12 by an uncle. His father had known what was happening but said nothing, accepting bottles of whisky from this uncle. Once the boys had grown up he disappeared. Michael would come around to the house frequently and became friends with our family. I told my wife all about his experiences some time after she had met him: she took to him and liked him – so much so that he occasionally came on family outings with us.

On one occasion we went by coach on a family trip to see the miniature Blue Railway. Michael was invited. But during the journey something happened which made my wife suspicious. Perhaps she saw the way he looked at me, or heard something we might have said to each other. She asked me if he was my lover. I admitted that he was and had been for some time.

There were tears from both of them; it was a very difficult time. Later I talked at length with her and told her I had done my best to go straight and what had been happening on my business trips, explaining the risks I was taking in public toilets. I tried to reassure her that since I had met him I was no longer doing that.

Instead of telling me to get out of the house – as she had every right to do – she reluctantly agreed that I should carry on seeing him. She said it was better that I should have Michael than every 'Tom, Dick and Harry'.

Michael continued to come around to the house. He was very unhappy at his home; his mother was ill and his father, by now bed-ridden, was permanently on a couch one of the only two rooms downstairs, and would demand that Michael buy him a bottle of whisky a day. If he did not get his drink he would try to hit Michael with the fireside poker. His brothers had left home and Michael felt he just had to stay to look after his mother.

Michael needed someone to talk to and he found he could talk to Vera about his troubles; she helped him and felt sorry for him. I managed to help by getting his mother into a home for a while. Then his father died, and instead of being relieved Michael was utterly distraught for some time.

Not surprisingly, Vera wanted to know exactly what Michael and I did together, so I told her in some detail. She didn't seem too shocked and, strange though it may seem, our family life carried on much as before. Once a week Michael would baby-sit for us while I took Vera out to a restaurant for dinner. Michael would stay the night sleeping on a put-u-up in the study. But one night, the strain of the situation became very apparent – and the true effects on Vera of my relationship with Michael emerged. After returning home, I was missing for a few minutes before bed: Vera asked where I had been. Without really thinking, I said, 'I've just been to kiss Michael goodnight.' Vera was distraught. She said, 'Oh you don't kiss him as well, do you?' It was as if she could cope with the knowledge that I was having sex with another man, but the thought that we were sharing the tenderness and intimacy of kissing was simply too much.

Michael was not naturally gay. He had been sexually abused as a small child and had been in a very unhappy home. He needed love and affection and was looking for it in public toilets when I meet him. As time wore on his mother came home; since the death of his father she had been a lot better. Then I discovered that Michael was meeting a girl. It hurt, but I encouraged him, knowing that he wanted to do what I had done – get married, settle down and have a family.

I approved of the first girl he met but the relationship didn't last and they broke up. It wasn't too long before he met someone else – and I had serious reservations about this new one. Sadly, these eventually proved to be well founded.

His new girlfriend was older than him with two small children; I thought she was on the lookout for a breadwinner, but Michael was smitten. He duly married her and they had a son of their own. A few years later he was lucky and won £2,000 on the football pools: it was a lot of money in those days and I was happy for him. We lost touch after his windfall until a friend told me he had left his wife. She had spent all the money, then kicked him out and he was now living rough in a squat and doing drugs.

It took some time but I tracked him down and helped him back on to his feet. It wasn't too long before we became lovers again, during which time he went to see a psychiatrist or counsellor of some kind who told him that his problems stemmed from his being abused as a child.

When Michael told me all this I felt guilty and wondered aloud about the effect and the propriety of our relationship. But he was adamant, saying: 'You have never ever done anything wrong as far as I am concerned. You are the only one that has ever helped me. You have loved me and were always there when I needed you.'

I often think of Michael, and of this conversation. It crystallised in my mind what a relationship is all about, whoever the relationship is with. Whether it is man and woman, man and man or woman and woman, a true relationship is a matter of love and of need – the real need of one person for another. And, whatever the sex or the orientation of the people involved, I wonder: what can be wrong with that?

For the record, Michael is now living happily with another woman. We are still great friends and not too long ago we met and, at his request, we managed to find a quiet spot for a kiss. He told me he still loves me.

And so the sixties ended. George Montague was now a well-established businessman with a thriving patternmaking company. I was also a loving and devoted father and, though it may sound conceited, performing truly valuable public services with the Scouts and disabled children.

But there was another George Montague: the homosexual man in a heterosexual marriage. A man whose sexual desires could no longer be buttoned down or safely brushed under the carpet. I was gay and I knew it. The problem was that others didn't – and that problem was about to turn my life upside down.

TEN

How, if you are old enough to have lived through it, do you remember 1974? The introduction of the three-day week (as a way to conserve electricity) in January? The murder of 11 people by Irish nationalists in the M62 bombing in February? It was a year of IRA terrorism, with bomb attacks on the Tower of London and in pubs in Birmingham and Guildford. Maybe you remember the fact that there were two general elections that year. Perhaps you recall, with a shudder, the seemingly inexorable rise of the National Front and the death of an anti-fascist protestor in demonstrations against it. Or the disappearance of Lord Lucan after the murder of his children's nanny.

I remember all of this and more. But I remember July 1974 with a pain that still lingers. Because that was the month when my world fell apart.

It was a summer's evening and I was in one of two cubicles in a public toilet. After the end of my relationship with Michael my urges had once again got the better of me and I had returned to the pleasures of cottaging. In the adjacent cubicle that night was a man in his 50s: I learned later that he was married with children – just like me in many respects. In the wall between the two cubicles there was a hole through which I could see him masturbating; I was doing the same. He then put his penis through the hole: he did not have an erection and I didn't touch it. Instead I continued with what Baden-Powell called self-abuse.

Suddenly there was a very loud bang on the locked door and a voice shouted: 'Open up! Police! Both of us were both arrested. One policeman had apparently been given a leg-up by his colleague to peer over the top of the cubicles. I looked at this officer: he was young, obsessively homophobic and I knew I was in trouble. Although I hadn't actually been doing anything illegal, I realised that this wouldn't stop the police. Sure enough, I was charged with the old and horrible offence of gross indecency. I would also soon discover that the young policeman lied in his evidence against me.

It had been seven years since Parliament had decriminalised homosexuality. But, if anything, the climate for gays was more dangerous than it had been before the change in the law. Police forces still targeted homosexual meeting places and gay bashing had entered the public lexicon. Packs of skinheads – often National Front supporters, for the two were frequently synonymous – would target homosexual men and kick them into unconsciousness for the perceived sin of being 'queer'. Outlandish though this may seem to us now, it's worth remembering that it would be another four years before homosexuals had an anthem of their own: *Glad To Be Gay* was then still unwritten, much less released.

And George Montague: who was he that summer of 1974? Still outwardly a conventional family man; and not, I think, just outwardly. Our children were young and I enjoyed family life very much. As soon as the children started to arrive I had shot cinefilm of every event from their birth onwards.

Every Boxing Day, because we had the biggest house, all my family would gather for the festive celebrations. After dinner we would all adjourn to my study-cum-cinema and enjoy the fruits of my domestic filming. This had become such a successful tradition that I bought a new camera, the latest model, and a new projector. I would spend many hours editing the raw footage and putting on more sound. Yes, George Montague was a family man – and loved it.

I was also a pillar of the community: such a strange phrase but one that is entirely accurate. Not only was I running a successful business, employing people and bringing work to a country that was rapidly diving into the misery of financial crises and unemployment, but I was also a decorated and dynamic Scout leader. I had brought together like-minded volunteers to create and run regular events for lads who, through their handicaps, would never otherwise have known this excitement.

And now, at the age of 51, I was about to be disgraced; to be exposed as a pervert, a man who committed disgusting acts with other men in public toilets.

Through my solicitor I briefed a barrister who informed me that if the case was heard before a bench of magistrates there was a big risk of being found guilty. Magistrates, after all, are laypeople from ordinary walks of life and they tended to believe police evidence as if it was the word of God, brought down from the mountains by Moses. But my counsel also advised that I stood an excellent chance of a not-guilty verdict if I insisted on trial in the higher Crown Court.

Here my case would be heard in front of a jury – men and women of my peers, 12 of them good and true. And although I had been in a public toilet, my co-accused and I were in separate cubicles with the doors closed and locked. It could, my barrister said, be argued that whatever I was doing, it was in private – and therefore not against the law. He also pointed out that the sole evidence against me was the word of a single policeman.

I gave his advice a great deal of thought. Plead guilty before the magistrates and hope the whole business would not be noticed? Or opt for a trial by jury, and an excellent chance of an acquittal? The question, a dilemma really, swamped my waking thoughts – and I was awake a lot with the worry of it.

In the end I chose not to exercise my right to a jury trial for one single, simple reason: to prevent the adverse publicity that would inevitably follow the evidence as it emerged in court. The words 'gross indecency' and 'a very well known Scout Commissioner' would have been the headlines, not only locally, but in all probability nationally, even if, as my counsel suggested, I was acquitted. Crown Court cases almost invariably attract much greater press attention than local magistrates' benches. The trial would be all over the evening papers to be discussed in pubs up and down the land. 'Mud sticks', as they say ('they' being the know-it-alls and busybodies who are only to happy to share their opinions loudly and widely), a phrase usually followed by 'there's no smoke without fire'.

And above all I was worried about what would undoubtedly be very bad publicity for the Scout movement. What, I could hear the prosecution barrister asking in my mind, was this respectable Scout leader – a man in charge of the nation's youth – doing in a public toilet about a mile from his home? What indeed.

Throughout my entire Scouting career I had believed in good publicity, and was very well known to the head reporters of the two local newspapers. I had given them both a great deal of material on all my Scouting activities over the years. And so I quietly talked to them both and explained the whole story. They were very sympathetic. I admitted that while I was dreading the publicity for my own sake and that of my family I was most concerned for the good name of Scouting. I explained that I had decided to go before the Magistrates – but I was damned if I was going to plead guilty to something I hadn't done.

My co-accused must have received different advice – or at least chosen a less hazardous course. He pleaded guilty (in fairness, he had poked his penis through the hole in the cubicle wall) and so his case came up a week or so before mine. There was a full report in both local papers that described his behaviour as having been 'with another man'. I wasn't named, but I felt very sorry for this man. His life would now be ruined. When my hearing came around I was horribly disappointed by the way the solicitor who represented me handled the proceedings. Because I was pleading not guilty my case came up after a succession of other short hearings. It was very late in the afternoon when I walked into the courtroom; I noticed there were no reporters there.

But my solicitor failed to fight the case with any vigour. He didn't challenge the police officer on his false testimony, nor bring out the officier's obvious homophobia. He did not call my co-accused as a witness to testify that I had not touched him or done anything that could constitute an act of gross indecency. He seemed most concerned about my refusal to have any character witnesses appear on my behalf. That in itself said a lot about his mindset – character witnesses generally only offer mitigating testimony, rather than anything that speaks of the innocence of the man in the dock.

As the barrister had predicted, I was found guilty. I was given a fine.

The following day I went to see one of the most senior officials of the Scouts in Berkshire. For very many years he had been a close personal friend. Both of us had lived a secret gay lifestyle before we got married to our respective wives. We had met long before he joined the Scout movement as an adult leader. At that time he and I had both been struggling with our sexuality, torn between the demands of conventional society and the (then illegal) desires to have sex with other men. Both of us had done the latter while trying to obey the former.

There was an additional irony in that at one time this man had helped me, as a layperson, with my Scout troop and had behaved in a way that could have caused him to be investigated. On the first night that he came to my troop meeting at the hospital, he sat on the side of the bed of one of the older boys holding his hand for some considerable time. I was extremely uncomfortable and told him I thought he ought to be careful about behaving in this way. Innocent or not, it could very easily be interpreted badly.

Surely, I thought to myself, if anyone in the Scouts knows what I'm going through it would be him. And it was in the capacity as a former gay friend rather than that of a senior Scouts official that I went to see him. I made it very clear to him that it was an unofficial 'off the record' visit.

I offered him my resignation and said I would leave it to him as to how and when I was quietly to leave the Scouts. Although it would have been on my police record, because there had – fortunately – been no publicity, no one else would have known or found out about my conviction. I explained that this was why I had not asked for any character witnesses because had my position in Scouting been put before the court then they also would have assumed that I would have been a danger to boys (which is what most people thought in those days, and many still do today) and the whole Scouting movement would have been tarnished.

Unfortunately my trust in this man proved to be misplaced. To be generous to him, I can only assume he thought that there was no possibility of keeping my conviction quiet, so he rang a retired County Commissioner for Scouts in another county (who lived nearby) and spilled the beans to him. Our private and off-the-record conversation was now destined to speed its way through the entire Scouts movement.

The upshot was that instead of resigning quietly at the most opportune time – for the Scouts and for me – I was dishonourably dismissed. All the most senior Scouters in any way connected with me were informed, and I had to hand over the leadership of the local Camp to one of them. I also had to return my warrant book to Headquarters and the leave the Scout movement for ever.

Even today I find it hard to express the hurt and betrayal I felt. I had given half a lifetime to the Scouting movement – sacrificing all of my free time (and much that was not really free). I had created, developed and brought to happy fruition camps for disabled youngsters who otherwise would never have enjoyed the Scouting life. I had run Gang Shows, raised money. In short, I had given more than a quarter of a century to an organisation I loved, believed in and whose trust – whatever the facts of my conviction – had never once betrayed.

Now I was forced to cut myself off from all members of the movement – both men and boys – and it hurt. It hurt terribly.

To make matters even worse I also heard through one of my closest friends that because there had been no publicity giving the facts of the case, when my former colleagues in the movement were told about my sudden and totally unexpected departure they were forced to assume that boys were involved.

There was nothing I could do except to cut myself off completely from everyone who had anything to do with Scouting. I was now not just a disgraced leader, a man who had sex with other men in public toilets – around me was the fatal, if utterly baseless, stench of paedophilia. It was terribly, terribly unfair: I had never had any desire at all for sex with boys, much less done anything to one in my charge.

But because I had been cast out – with all the rumours and innuendo that provoked – I was completely unable to defend myself or deny the vicious whisperings.

I was however – in this as in much else – lucky to have the support of Vera. We talked the whole business over. She, of course, had to know the full gory detail of what had happened. But with her blessing and backing we kept it from everybody else. With the exception of my wife, none of my family – not my parents, nor my children – or any of my employees or my customers, ever knew of my conviction. For that, at that time I was very thankful.

But the treachery by my former friend rankled terribly. It ate away inside me. He had betrayed my confidence, and even though I had assured him that I would ring him and inform him the moment I heard that there might be any publicity, he had reported me in the sure and certain knowledge of what would happen. He made a grave mistake and I was very deeply hurt that he should have made the matter of my private visit to him and my trouble known to others without speaking to me first or waiting to hear from me whether or not I had been successful in avoiding publicity. And it was doubly painful to know that this had been done by a man who, like me, had also enjoyed sex with other men.

I had, unquestionably, been let down by someone from within the homosexual world. It would not, sadly, be the last time that the gay community betrayed its own – not for me and not for others like me.

ELEVEN

Acquiring a criminal record drastically changed my life. I felt that I had a genuine reason to be angry about my conviction for gross indecency. In the first place it was a discriminatory piece of otherwise victimless legislation that could only be levelled at gays; and secondly, while I had on many occasions undoubtedly been guilty of sexual activity in public toilets, ironically on this occasion I was innocent.

Being forced out of the Scouts, a movement to which I had given 53 years, man and boy, felt like a bereavement. There was a huge, aching hole in my life. I missed the camaraderie and I worried about who, if anyone, would now ensure that disabled lads had the same Scouting chances as their able-bodied brothers.

But in time I came to see that there was an upside. Being excommunicated – especially so brutally – finally set me free from my addiction to Scouting. And without its constant demands I found that I was able to spend much more time with my family – something that brought me (and, I hope, them) great comfort and immense pleasure. Nonetheless, there was something missing. I found that much of the attraction of Scouting had been the constant solving of problems and fighting battles for those less fortunate than me. I needed a new campaign to fight.

Happily, when one door closes another opens. Very soon after I was forced to resign, a friend of mine approached me and told me he had bought a sailing yacht in kit form. He was now facing the daunting task of putting all the bits together and had realised he needed assistance. He knew I was a woodworker and asked me if I would help him with the tricky woodwork involved.

It was a request that would, in time, lead me to discover the twin joys of restoring a boat and then taking it proudly out of harbour under sail.

Nothing on a boat is straight or square, and everything has to be individually fitted. I found the work a complete relaxation, much-needed time away from my business and from the family. I enjoyed it so much that I started to seriously think about fitting out a boat of my own.

Living near the Thames I had, as a boy and young man, done a lot of messing about in boats, but my only experience of getting under sail was once taking out a 'pram dinghy' – a small starter-type craft – for half an hour while the family were off shopping. The little boat was very sturdy, but it seemed to have an enormous amount of sail for its size – about 10 square feet of yellow mackintosh-type material. After two near capsizes, when I thought the boat would sink and I would face the ignominy of have to swim back without it, I managed to get back to the shore. It gave me my first and vital lesson about the raw power of even a light wind on a relatively small sail.

Following the launch of my friend's boat I had got the bug. Not for sailing but for fitting out a boat. This time I knew I had to involve the family. My daughter Paula was 13, Martin 12 and Edward 11. We decided we would buy a boat, fit it out and then if we didn't like sailing we could sell it at a profit. We all went down to a marina to look at what was available. Paula said she felt seasick on the pontoon. My wife did not say much, but the boys were all for it.

We were invited down to a friend's boat for the weekend; it was moored some way out on a swinging mooring in Langstone Harbour. My wife and daughter were relieved that the boat was only big enough for four so they did not have to come. We loaded up everything that was required: I was amazed how much *stuff* seemed to be needed for sailing. We all got into a small dinghy and rowed out to the boat: the two boys had life jackets on, and before we got halfway I wished I had one too, as the water was very choppy.

We were supposed to spend a whole lovely weekend on the water, the aim being to give me and my sons a taste for the sailing life. As it turned out the only pleasant part of the weekend was the Friday evening. Still safely on our mooring, with us all well fed and the boys asleep in their bunks, my friend and I poured ourselves 'sundowners' in the cockpit. But that night the wind got up to force eight and stayed there for 30 hours. With no possibility of getting ashore and no way to contact anyone, we were stuck on a craft so small that I couldn't even stand up straight in the cabin.

We did attempt to put to sea, and carefully inched the nose of the boat just outside the harbour entrance, but it was far too rough. There was nothing for it but to sit tight and wait until the wind calmed down enough for us to row back to the shore.

I learned a valuable lesson that weekend and decided that if we were going to take up sailing it would have to be in a boat that I could stand up in. I was also determined that it would be fully equipped and something that we could afford to keep in a marina on a pontoon, so that we could step on and off with all the facilities that a teenage family would need.

And so *Woody* came into our lives. After visiting many boatyards to work out what type of boat would be best, our decision came down to a 26-foot Westerly Centaur, or a 27-foot Marcon Sabre. I visited both yards and was shown all stages of production. I was impressed by the sturdiness and the layout of the Sabre. It was more expensive, but as luck would have it they had one they'd had for some time. The person who ordered it didn't like the colour – phantom grey. I thought the colour was about the least important aspect. In fact, I liked it, but said I didn't, and got £500 off the asking price – no small sum in 1976.

By this time my parents had moved into a smaller property on the same estate. Adjoining their house was a barn with a hayloft and a door 10 feet from the ground, into which the hay was once unloaded straight from the horse-drawn wagons. I asked their permission to have the boat delivered there.

The budget kit was delivered in December 1976, on a trailer towed by a Land Rover. The keel was only about six inches from the ground. Two lorry jacks lowered her onto a piece of two-inch-thick plywood. I realised the weight of the boat when this bent and sank into what had been Dad's beautifully tended lawn. We put some wooden props around to hold her up, and within half an hour there she was with the cockpit level with, and a couple of feet away from, the loft door.

The loft was already set up as a workshop and over the next two and a half years I spent on average 20 hours a week working on her with help from family and friends. During the two winters I attended a Yacht Masters training course, then two annual holidays in chartered boats. What I learned from them proved invaluable in the fitting out.

Where did I get all my tips? I read everything I could lay my hands on, yachting magazines and books, talked to other sailors and visited the London Boat Show every year.

It was now May 1978, well into the sailing season. There were many other jobs still to do but I was now impatient – I wanted to get her afloat. I wanted my mother to name and launch her, but the second bit proved too difficult to arrange so we concentrated on the naming ceremony. Mum stood on an upturned crate, which served as a podium, then, with a half-bottle of sparkling wine, she christened our *Woody*.

After that it was just a question of getting *Woody* down to our chosen mooring at Brighton Marina, where I could carry on working on her in the water. Brighton turned out to be an auspicious choice in many ways – and not all of them were good.

I knew by now that I was gay – and gay for life. I was, of course, still married to Vera and we still shared the family home. But she had, like me, come to accept that my sexual desires were for men not women, and our marriage became more of a friendship – a close and loving one – than a conventional relationship.

It was on one of my trips to Brighton Marina that I met the man who would become my fourth long-term lover. And, as ever, there were as many tears as there was laughter in the seven years our relationship lasted.

I first saw Steve across a lively bar in Brighton one lunchtime. He was extremely good looking and I was attracted to him straight away. He was also, usefully, with someone I knew, so I asked to be introduced. Equally fortunately, it turned out that our mutual friend was just that – he wasn't, as I suddenly feared, Steve's partner.

We sat and talked for a long time and Steve told me that he was 20 years old: his English sounded a little strange and he explained that he had recently come back to England from Germany where his parents lived. His mother was German and his father was a former British soldier.

I asked him where he was staying, and he surprised me by saying nowhere: 'I slept under the pier last night.' Instantly I was on my guard. I was worried that he might be a rent boy. But as our chat continued, it became clear that he wasn't a male prostitute – simply someone outgoing, cheerful and who took life as it came: he didn't seem to have a care in the world.

I spent the rest of the afternoon with him, weighing him up and finding out more about him. He said he didn't know whether he was gay or straight. He had had a boyfriend in Germany; he had a row with his parents and left home; he was looking for a job and somewhere to stay; he didn't seem to know much about the British system of social security. I invited him to stay on the boat for the night and said I would help him sort himself out in the morning. That night I took him to a gay club, but when we got to the door the doorman, who knew me, held up his hand to stop us: 'You can come in George, but not him.'

Apparently on a previous occasion Steve had hit someone who had tried it on with him. As a result we returned for the night to the boat, where I put him in the fore cabin while I slept in the saloon. In the morning he said: 'You are the first bloke I've been back with who didn't try anything.' I could feel the beginnings of trust developing.

In the morning I helped him as I'd promised. I had the use of a small room by arrangement with a sailing friend; he was prepared to let Steve use it. I left, telling Steve I would see him the following weekend. When we met up again as arranged he told me that jobs were very difficult to find in Brighton: it was winter and out of season on the coast. As I was working on *Woody* I asked him if he wanted to help me with the project, for which I would pay him. He jumped at the chance and turned out to be a very good worker.

The more I got to know Steve the more I liked him. I was also attracted to him, but, mindful of what he had said on that first night, I did nothing about it. Then, one day, I met someone I fancied and who fancied me. I took him back with me. I explained to Steve and asked him to clean the car while we were inside for half an hour or so. When I emerged afterwards I discovered that both Steve and the car had gone. I cursed my stupidity: 'What a fool I am. I thought I was such a good judge of character.'

I went down to the police station giving details of the car and explaining to the officers that there was a possibility Steve would make for Dover, and then head back to Germany on a ferry. With that, the telephone on the desk rang – it was my new friend to tell me that Steve had returned.

Relief flooded in, but just as quickly ebbed away. I realised that Steve had no licence or insurance – and that I'd reported him missing with my car. I looked at the policeman. He said: 'Tell him to come down here – but not in the car.' I sat down to wait, head in my hands and wishing I had waited longer before going to the police. Steve soon arrived, sporting a large grin. I was furious, and told him in no uncertain terms that he was in deep and serious trouble.

At which point my estimation of Her Majesty's Constabulary shot up a few notches. The policeman questioned Steve carefully, told him he had been very foolish and spelled out what would have happened had he been involved in an accident or stopped by a patrol car. And then he simply told him never to do it again.

I was astonished. I asked: 'Aren't you going to charge him?' The policeman smiled. 'No,' he said. 'Fortunately for him we didn't see him.' And that was that. Considering my past brushes with the law, I considered that, all in all, we had been remarkably fortunate. On the way back I asked Steve why he had done it. Calm as you like, he told me that he had been jealous. From that day on we became lovers and would be together for almost exactly seven years.

I told Steve there was a much better chance of getting a job in Slough and he duly moved up there. He stayed in a social security hostel and very quickly found jobs. Employers were very impressed to find that he spoke fluent German and gradually our life settled into a happy pattern – we spent most weekends in Brighton, sailing or working on *Woody*.

But life – or at least my life – never runs smoothly for very long. The first indication of choppy waters ahead came in a gay bar on the Brighton seafront. It wasn't, though, an exclusively homosexual haunt; many straight people would call in and probably never noticed that it was gay. One day Steve was chatting to two good-looking girls: the chatting up was evidently being done more by them than Steve, and finally he told them that he was gay and that I was his boyfriend.

Their immediate comment was: 'What a waste!' ('What a cheek!' was my reaction). Then they said: 'Are all these chaps in here gay?' When we explained that most of the clientele were indeed homosexual, the girls were astonished. 'But they don't look gay,' they protested. I sighed. I had heard this reaction so often from the general public. They all thought that gays were very obvious and camp, like Quentin Crisp, John Inman – then playing the effeminate shop assistant in the hit television show *Are You Being Served* – or (worse) Dick Emery and Larry Grayson. These characters were, like most homosexual people portrayed on TV in those days, very camp. And in turn, most straight people thought all gays were really like that.

It wasn't a terribly serious incident and nothing else came of it. But in retrospect it was a clear example of the casual and unthinking pressures which heterosexual people often visit on homosexuals: the idea that an attractive man should be lost to the feminine half of the country seems somehow to be perceived as either an affront or a challenge. It also, though I couldn't have known it that day, presaged what would eventually happen with Steve.

The second event was much more serious – very much more serious indeed. And, once again, it involved the police.

It was early spring and I was working on the boat when a young voice from the gangway above called out: 'Can I help yer, mister?' I looked up and there was a young lad. I asked who he was and what he wanted. He told me that his name was Trevor; he was 16 and would be leaving school in the summer and so was looking for casual work.

There is always a lot of work that needs to be done on a boat at the end of the winter season. I had installed a huge amount of woodwork on *Woody* (hence the name), all of which needed attention. And so I told him he could help out with the varnishing and rubbing down. He was a good worker and we got on well together. Over the next few weeks he would sometimes already be at the boat, hard at his labours, by the time I arrived.

Over the years I have had several helpers who do work in return for a day's sailing. But these casual labourers were unreliable and, as often as not, wanted to bring their mates along and always started to muck about. Trevor wasn't like that. After a while he asked if he could stay the night on the boat. Of course I said no. He was still a young lad and would have needed his parents' permission. I didn't want to get into that; I had in the back of my mind how easily this could be misinterpreted.

Then, on the weekend before the Easter holidays I told him I was going out for the first sail of the season. I was heading down to Newhaven for the weekend with another friend. Trevor pleaded with me to let him come, saying his parents would not mind and that they knew he had been helping me.

Foolishly, I gave in. I told him that I could not get down until the Saturday as I had a singing engagement the night before, but that he could come down on the Good Friday and finish off the work on the boat. I showed him where I had a spare key hidden. I also explained that as we would not be sailing until the afternoon we would have time for me call in on his parents and get their permission for the weekend of sailing.

As it turned out my friend cancelled at the last minute and so that Saturday I arrived on my own. I found Trevor sitting in the cockpit with a big smile on his face: 'I've finished all the work,' he said proudly, and I could see right away that it did indeed look as if he had done a lot. As often happened the sea was too rough to think about going out that afternoon, but as the forecast was better for the next day I told him we could go tomorrow. When I got inside *Woody* I noticed that the waste bin was full. I always kept a lot of tinned food on board and casually expressed surprise to Trevor about the amount he had managed to eat in one day. But I thought no more about it.

Then two men appeared alongside *Woody*. I knew straight away they were policemen. They immediately spoke to Trevor, asking him to confirm his surname. By now, Trevor looked very guilty; he gave the officers his details and was told to get off the boat immediately. Before I had a chance to ask what was happening, the second policeman stepped onto the boat, went down into the cabin and started poking around. I followed him and asked what Trevor had done – and what he was doing rummaging through my boat without any invitation.

His only response was to ask me to confirm my name. And then he said: 'I am arresting you on suspicion of child abduction and abuse.'

I couldn't believe my ears. I had never laid a finger on Trevor – much less kidnapped him as the officer seemed to be suggesting. But at the back of my mind a small, nagging voice said: 'Here we go again. Another police fit-up.'

Apparently Trevor had been on the boat all of the previous week without telling me or his parents; they had, not unreasonably, reported him missing. One of the marina staff had heard a report about a missing boy; he had seen Trevor on the boat a day or two before and on that Saturday morning he contacted the police. They had asked him for details of the owner: on checking my name against the Criminal Records Office database they discovered that I had a conviction for gross indecency. They put what they assumed was two and two together – convicted homosexual with runaway boy on his boat must equal predatory paedophile. I was taken to Brighton Police Station.

What happened to me there was utterly humiliating. I was told to strip: swabs were taken from my penis, anus and mouth. Then I was put into a cell and left alone there for more than four hours. Finally two detectives came in: one of them attempted to browbeat me, by accusing me – in a very loud voice – of sexually abusing Trevor.

They said they had all the evidence, that they had examined my waste bin and the boat and found what they wanted. They also told me that they had medically examined Trevor and that he was at that moment in another room, in floods of tears and had confessed 'everything'. I couldn't believe what they were saying. I had done absolutely nothing to Trevor: how could he have confessed to something I hadn't done? All I could do was deny – vehemently – that I had ever touched him.

The detectives kept me locked up for another four hours then, without charging me, I was released on police bail. I was to report back in one week. It was late at night and I was in my working clothes without a penny on me. When I explained this to the detectives, expecting that at the very least I would be taken back to the boat, they shrugged and said, 'hard luck'. I had to walk the mile back to my *Woody*.

On the Easter Sunday Trevor arrived on the gangway. I was not pleased to see him and when I had finished telling him how much trouble he had caused, I put him in the car and told him to direct me to his home. On the way he told me how sorry he was; that he had run away from home before and no one had ever cared or reported it. He told me that the police had done to him the same that they did to me, telling him that I had confessed and told them everything. He said that he told them: 'You lot are bloody liars; you bring him here and let me hear him say that'. A fat lot of good that did either of us.

When we arrived at his house I was astonished by his parents' reaction. I had assumed they would be furious about Trevor staying on the boat. I think in their position – and had it been one of my sons who had disappeared from home – I would have had a few strong words to say. But they didn't seem to care and didn't seem to want to listen to anything I had to say, so I left reflecting on how strange some people can be.

I was due to appear back at the police station a week later, so I asked around and was put in touch with a lady solicitor who was a lesbian. On the way down to the station she asked me about Trevor and what he had said. When I told her he had said nothing, for we had done nothing, she shocked me. 'You're very lucky that he's such a good lad. Usually the police bully the kids into saying something happened even when it didn't.' Perhaps I was naïve, but I was appalled. Arresting or even fitting up gay men for cottaging in public toilets was one thing, but for the police deliberately to have men falsely branded as paedophiles was disgusting.

When we arrived at the station the detectives told me they were not charging me with any offence. Inwardly I was seething: 'I should think not: there never had been any offence – just your own vile prejudice.' But I kept my thoughts to myself as they handed me back all the items that they had taken from the boat.

It had been, as my solicitor explained, a very nasty run-in. I told Trevor to stay away from the boat, but he continued to come down to the marina: I would find him waiting for me, not on the boat but in the car park. So one day – and in full public view – we sat down and had a heart-to-heart talk. He told me that he was gay and that he had been going with men since he was 14. He also told me that he had been informed I was homosexual, and that he'd known that when he approached me for work. Then he told me that he was in love with me. It was not what I wanted to hear.

By this time he had left school and was 17. But I firmly told him that the age of consent was 21, and that I would go to prison if I had any sort of sexual relationship with him. I spelled out that if there was even a sniff of something improper the police would be out to get us – and I reminded him of the very unpleasant examinations that we had both been put though at the police station.

I also gave him the fruits of my experience of half a

century on the planet: it was, I told Trevor, very possible that he might not be gay, that I had known of quite a number of lads who had started having sex with men as young as 14 but who had turned out to be straight in the end. These were often boys from unhappy homes, or those in council homes, and the phase they were going through was to do with the need to be wanted and receive affection. (As it happened, in Trevor's case I was completely right on this score: he eventually found a girl and got married.)

And finally, for good measure, I told him that I was still in love with Steve. And that was true, too – for good or ill.

TWELVE

The eighties have a lot to answer for.

It was in this decade that the world caught up with the gay scene, and not in a good way. For some time – a reaction perhaps to the liberation which had flowed from the decriminalisation of homosexual activity – the scene in many cities across Britain had been one of unbridled hedonism. Perhaps this is what led to a backlash against us when Aids first appeared. Certainly the disease helped foster the idea that homosexual men are promiscuous.

It is, as I've already noted, an accusation that puzzles me. I've been gay all my life and have, perhaps, an unrivalled position from which to view the history of our little sub-culture: I certainly don't know any other gay men happily and healthily progressing towards their 100th birthday. The best explanation – other than lingering prejudice – that I've come up with is that some of us are less jealous and possessive than the heterosexual world – or at least than straight people likes to believe they are. Which brings us back to Steve.

On very many levels, the early 1980s were a difficult time for me. It was during this time, a period when Steve and I were still lovers in a loving relationship, that my mother became very ill. I was very upset and worried about Mum so I saw a great deal less of Steve; I think too that perhaps that I didn't communicate with him well enough as the months wore on.

And so, one day I received a telephone call to tell me that he was in hospital. He had taken an overdose. He had been put on a stomach pump and had nearly died. And although the doctors were sure he would pull through, he was still very ill. It also quickly became clear that this was more than an attention-seeking attempt: in addition to my absences, Steve was having great problems with his parents, who had come over to England to live.

Steve had a love-hate relationship with his mother. They were both very much alike and they both had a problem with nerves. Being forced together only exacerbated the tension, but the last straw for him was, apparently, that he thought I didn't want him any more.

As was routine in cases of attempted suicide he was referred for psychiatric assessment at the Windsor Hospital. By this time I knew Steve better than anyone alive, including his parents. I knew that at this difficult point in time he needed me and indeed we needed each other. I was prepared to do anything that was best for him: and so I went with him to see the psychiatrist.

We were briefly seen together and then I was told to leave

the room. Soon after Steve came storming out and shouted: 'That idiot wants me to leave you!' So much for sympathetic mental health services.

I decided to get Steve out of the hostel where he was living. I saw an advert for a room in Windsor. Mother was frequently in and out of the hospital there, so I rented it. The room was at the very top of a large old Victorian house and it had a beautiful view of the castle from the window. The landlady told me that the house used to belong to Queen Victoria's personal physician.

Steve smoked very heavily. He knew I hated it and he promised me he would try to give it up. But I said we had to plan it and only do it when the time was right and he was ready. With a magic marker I wrote out on one of those yellow sticky-strip pads all the 'bad' words I could think of to do with cigarettes: unhealthy, dirty, smelly, expensive and very many more besides. I stuck them all over the walls.

Finally, the big day came: the day he would quit for good. He had his last cigarette after breakfast and then I took down all the cards and put up dozens more with words such as, healthy, clean, sweet-smelling. He lasted until lunchtime then he started to sweat: he was going cold turkey. But I found that if I could talk him out of having one for one minute, then he was okay for another hour or so. And then I would take him for long runs in Windsor Great Park, which was close by.

But try as I might, the nicotine addiction was just too strong: Steve managed four days before it got the better of him: he swore at his manager and walked out of work to find the nearest tobacconist. He is still a heavy smoker.

Mum, meanwhile, was getting worse. For about the

previous 10 years my parents had lived in a small bungalow looking on to a pleasant garden, which Dad kept busy maintaining and improving. The first indication that something was wrong had been the death of their beloved black Labrador bitch. Mum and Bess were devoted and every day would take her for long walks. But after Bess died (at the advanced age of 17) Mum gradually changed. She stopped going for long walks, saying there was now no need. Then one day Dad said to me: 'There's something wrong with your mother son, she has become very forgetful: she's giving me egg and bacon for every meal.'

My wife and I had a look around Mum's kitchen and found there was nothing in the larder but eggs, bacon and marmalade. With the help of my sister-in-law, my wife and I managed to humour Mother and, without upsetting her, ensure that they both had proper meals. But as time passed we noticed that often when we said something to her, Mum would simply smile and say something in reply which didn't make any sense. The doctor arranged for her to have a brain scan: the diagnosis was that her brain at the front of her head had shrunk: Alzheimer's. It was the first time any of us had ever heard or read of it. She spent some time in Windsor Hospital, never questioning us or getting upset. I visited her every day, sometimes twice a day, combining the trips with time spent with Steve.

In the end she was sent home – something that proved a serious worry for Dad. She would turn on the gas stove then forget to light it; when she started going for walks again she would fail to come home and we would find her half a mile away when it was getting dark, sitting on a seat by the roadside.

We had a family conference at which we decided we would do all we could not to put her into a home. I would sleep there and the others would do shifts during the day. Inevitably, the shift arrangement did not work for very long: everybody had their own family commitments and Mother was getting increasingly more difficult to look after (but never aggressive and rarely upset). She was in a world of her own for most of the time; we had lost the mother we all knew and loved.

The time came when we had no alternative but to put her into a private nursing home. I visited her every day: it was very terribly distressing because she was very unhappy and constantly cried, asking me to take her home.

She did have periods of lucidity, and it was during one of the moments when she was almost her old self that I tackled a family mystery. I had discovered from going though her private papers that she and father had not married until I was three years old. I asked her directly, Was Dad my father? I reassured her that I didn't mind in the least if he was not. He had always treated me just the same as my brothers and sisters and, even if he was not my actual parent, he was just as much a father to me, and much more so than the real one. Mum just cried and shook her head. 'You must ask your father, my dear.' I think then that I had my answer.

Not long before her 82nd birthday Mum was taken back into hospital. On the great day itself I collected her and took her home, sat her in the sitting room so that, one by one, all the family greeted her. She had 10 grandchildren by then and she named each one as they wished her happy birthday. Then Vera and I took her back to the hospital where she had been given a small room all to herself. We tucked her up in bed with all the cards around her. The nurses came in and sang happy birthday.

At seven o'clock the next morning the telephone rang; it was the sister to tell me that Mum had died during the night. She was as old as the century: it was 1982.

Mum's death was the catalyst for long overdue change. A few months later Vera and I talked and we realised that it was time to live apart. She knew, of course, about Steve (as she had known about my previous lovers), and perhaps she realised that with Mum gone I needed him more than ever. If we sold the house there would be enough for both of us to find new homes. But, of course, there was one step to take first: I had to come out to my children.

It was inevitably a horribly sad day. We had a little family meeting in which I plucked up my courage and said: 'I'm sorry guys, but you need to know that your dad is gay.' What shocked me most were not the tears, it was what Paula said: 'Oh, Dad, we've known for years.'

Some years earlier I had decided that where my sexuality was concerned I should try not to shock my children if it could be avoided. The decision had been prompted by Martin finding a copy of *Gay News* while he was earning his pocket money cleaning my car. He took it straight to his mother who told him to ask me about it. I had told him no direct lies: I said some of my best friends were gay and that I wanted to know more about them, and that if people in general knew more about them there would not be so much anti-gay prejudice. At the time there were numerous programmes on television about gays and sometimes plays with homosexuals in lead roles. I always wanted to watch them and when the children asked me why (they probably wanted to watch something else at the time) I told them the same thing: I wanted to know more about my friends' lifestyles. Now, after all the efforts I had make not to shock them, here was my eldest daughter taking the wind out of my sails by blithely reassuring me they had known my secret for years.

Vera and I decided not to divorce, but I moved into a small three-bedroomed house in Slough. I got it very cheaply as it needed a great deal of work doing; I put in central heating, rewired the whole place and completely redecorated inside and out. It was a relief to have my own space after such a long and unconventional marriage. And, of course, Steve was now able to live with me. It felt good, very good.

The person who suffered most during all these difficult days was my dad. Mum had always managed everything, made all the decisions, done everything except the garden. He was devoted to her and she to him. With her gone, Dad went downhill very quickly. He stopped doing the garden, saying: 'There's no one to do it for now.' I visited him at some time every day, often sitting with him for many hours in the evening mulling over happier times.

It was constantly on my mind to ask him if he was my real father. He had no idea I knew about the marriage certificate. But he was so unhappy that I was never able to bring myself to ask him. Mum's cryptic response was as close as I was ever going to get.

During mother's illness and in the months after her death Vera would, several times a week, walk more than two miles to take Dad his dinner and then I would drive over to bring her home. On one terrible day I was unable to do so and neither was I able to visit him that night. The next day when

Vera took his dinner over she found him sitting in his chair, his head on his chest with the empty dinner plate placed neatly on the floor at his side. He had died of a heart attack – but we knew it was really a broken heart. It was less than a year after Mum had passed away.

Mum had requested that she be cremated and we had kept her ashes in a little casket. Dad was buried in the family grave above my brother and grandmother. Mother's casket was placed on top of Dad's coffin.

The little churchyard and church at Hitcham is about as beautiful a spot as you could find, overlooking the great park with which we were all so familiar. Dad had for some years looked after the boiler for heating the church and had the very difficult job of cutting the grass around the graves. I used to help him sometimes, as well as being in the choir, both man and boy, a bellringer and server. I was very familiar with every detail and almost every grave. Together he and I would see if we could find the oldest gravestone, and we had discovered that many of them had eroded away and the inscriptions were no longer legible. I vowed there and then that the Montague family gravestone would always be readable.

I had the names of Grandmother, Brother Edward, Mother and Father engraved in bronze and mounted on a piece of Italian marble. It just gives the dates of birth and death. Underneath we inscribed my Christian name and those of my brother and two sisters – and the words: 'See you later.'

Steve was an enormous comfort to me during this difficult year, and the house in Slough became an integral part of the local gay scene, with parties and barbeques – *bar-be-queers* as we took to calling them – all summer long. But it was at a barbeque given by one of the members of our gay sailing club that I came – unexpectedly – face to face with my namesake: Lord Edward Montagu – Peer of The Realm and once detained in Her Majesty's Prison for the terrible sin of loving another man.

The party was at a beautiful house near his Lordship's ancestral home of Beaulieu. Later on in the evening I went up to Lord Edward explaining that I wanted to introduce myself because we had several things in common. 'We are both about the same age. We are both married. Both have the same number of children. We are both yacht owners and sailors. We're both gay and are both named Montague – although, unlike you, I have an "e" on the end of my name.'

I told him that I had known of him ever since his trial and imprisonment, that all gays had followed his misfortune, buying not one but several papers and reading every word. And I said how grossly unfair and unjust it all had been and that he and his co-defendants all ought to receive a public apology.

But Lord Edward simply smiled: he said he had managed to 'live it down' and that he did not want to be a professional victim. It would not be until 50 years after the infamous trial that this quiet, dignified man would speak of the torment he endured. I admired him greatly.

He was friendly and we chatted for some time: his Lordship told me that we would be related (at least somewhere, somehow in the dim and distant past) and that our family name originated from Normandy. Then Steve joined us and I introduced him as my partner, at which point we were invited to visit Lord Montagu at Palace House, Beaulieu.

I have to say that it crossed my mind that his Lordship might have found Steve rather attractive, and that this was the reason for our invitation. I couldn't say I blamed him – Steve was a very attractive man. And there's that difference between the gay and the straight worlds: I suspected there was a slight twinkle in Lord Edward's eye – but I wasn't remotely jealous.

On the day of our visit His Lordship personally showed us around, including parts of his Palace not normally seen by the public. Then he said: 'George why don't you go and fetch your car? Drive it around the block to the front door while I show Steve some more of the house.' I smiled inwardly and thought to myself, 'Told you so.'

Beaulieu is a vast estate and it was about half an hour before I returned with the car. I must say I enjoyed driving through his impressive entrance gates and up to the stately front door. I sat in the car and waited until they appeared, Lord Edward's arm protectively around Steve's shoulder. I took a photograph.

As I have said, I am not the jealous or possessive type, but even if I were I need not have worried, for I am positive Steve never let any other man touch him from the day I met him, Baron or no Baron. But that didn't mean he was only having sex with me. Throughout our time together there were periods when Steve was also going out regularly with his girlfriend. At those times he stopped coming down to the boat with me.

Because, yes, Steve, like John and Michael before him, had a girlfriend. And because I loved him I encouraged him. Her name was Melanie and he brought her around to the house and then asked if she could stay on the weekends that I went down to the boat. Often I would come home and she was still there. Then one Sunday evening I put my hand into my dressing gown pocket and there was a pair of her knickers: it was the beginning of the end.

Melanie, of course, knew all about our relationship, but I think she thought that Steve would one day leave me for her. With a heavy heart I told Steve that she deserved him more than I did, and that he would be so much better off with her than me: she could give him the acceptance which comes with a heterosexual relationship. And she could give him children.

Poor Steve. He was torn because he wanted us both. But it couldn't last and one evening all three of us went out to dinner: I told Steve that we must finish; the time had come to part. There were tears all round, but – with sadness and, I think, reluctance – he agreed. I was once again on my own.

THIRTEEN

When I got home on the night I parted with Steve, I had one thought and one thought only: 'What have I done?' It was one of the most miserable moments of my life: I was 65 – old enough to be a pensioner – separated from my wife and now back living alone.

And death was beginning to stalk me. First Mum, then Dad had passed away – traumatic times for anyone who loved his parents. But even more painfully Rodney, my very first lover, had also died.

I had always kept in touch with Rod. He had visited me often and one day he brought with him several pieces of furniture that we had made together, some with the tapestry on it that we had spent so many happy hours doing. We had originally divided these between us back when I got married and he had bought his first house. Initially I was reluctant to take his share from him – after all, we had made them together and they were physical embodiments of our memories of the precious years we had spent together. But he had insisted, telling me that he had a boyfriend in America and was going to see him for a month; he also mentioned that he might be going to live out there.

Reluctantly, I agreed. I said goodbye to him and wished him well. I didn't realise that would be the last time I'd see him. It was 1984 when I heard of his passing. I was at home when I got a telephone call from the man who had rented Rodney's house in England. He had received a phone call from America to say that Rod had died of a heart attack: he was just 48.

It took six weeks to get his ashes back from the States, but when they arrived we gave Rodney a proper send-off: there were about 200 people at the funeral. My wife came with me – despite the fact that she knew we had a relationship for some years before we were married she had always been very fond of him. But then that was Rodney: he was a very popular person.

At the funeral, his brother told me that Rodney had been warned by his doctors some years before that he was very ill; they had told him to stop working, stop having sex and to live the life of an invalid. But Rod told his brother that he would rather die than do that, and carried on just as normal. He told no one but his brother and no one else knew or suspected anything was wrong. It was then that I knew why he had given me back those things that he must have treasured.

Rodney's ashes had come back from America in a very well-made bronze box. After we had scattered them over his mother's grave, the question arose as to what to do with the box. I immediately asked if I could have it: I built it into a waterfall feature in the garden of my house.

Rodney left only one other item, besides his will. It was a letter, and it was addressed to me.

My dearest Monty,

You will only read this letter when I am no longer here. You may ask yourself 'Why?' I can only say I wanted you to know. It would be wrong to say I loved you from the moment I first saw you. But certainly soon after knowing you I realised I loved you and have continued loving you ever since. No one else ever really came into my life because no one could fill adequately the ideal you had created.

Knowing you intimately for so many years, years that were important because they were formative ones, gave me a standard to live up to and an ability to calmly accept compromise in life that was at least not easy. The years spent with you were unquestionably the happiest I have ever know, certainly enough to sustain me for the years I didn't have you, yet you had become so much a part of me that I was never truly without you.

The joy of your children pleased me and the happiness you had from your 'friend' made me happy, to close is difficult, all I can say is thank you for being who you are, and for knowing me.

God bless you. Roddy

That had been four years ago, but Rodney's letter had always brought me solace and comfort, just as he had done in life. Now, as I recovered from the parting from Steve, it helped me realise that I must carry on.

By that time business was becoming less easy. I had started the company in 1949 and we had survived some of the most turbulent economic times in modern history: inflation, recessions, three-day weeks and seemingly endless cycles of boom and bust. We now employed 32 men altogether, the largest Pattern Shop in the south of England at that time. The men regularly did 10 hours or so overtime and were very unhappy if this was stopped when we slackened off. But our main customers were the larger foundries: they were becoming more automated and the smaller ones were closing. We moved into smaller premises – the sale of my old industrial workshop realising a pleasant quantity of cash. But business was still difficult: it meant that we had to look further afield for work from customers. I had been required to travel abroad a great deal, and on several occasions had been to Pakistan. I could not have known it, but, in the aftermath of my break-up with Steve, some of the cultural problems of that troubled country were about to walk into my life.

I had decided on retail therapy as a way to salve the pain of missing Steve. I went to Harrods, spent a lot of money and then walked the mile or so to a gay pub in Soho. I sat facing the door still feeling, and I'm sure looking, fed-up. Then I looked up and saw, filling the doorway and smiling the smile that only Asians have, Hussein looking straight at me. He was almost 20, very slim and very good-looking.

We began chatting, and he told me that he was from Birmingham, an assertion which, given his accent, I readily believed. He told me some of his life story: he said he had known he was gay since his early teens, and that he'd had several lovers since leaving school. When his father said it was time for him to think about getting married he had told his father that he was gay. In some Muslim families this would elicit a very hostile response, but Hussein's father shrugged and said: 'So what? What had being gay got to do with it? It doesn't have to stop you getting married.'

Hussein hadn't seen it that way: he had left home and had been living for some time with an older man named Bob. But then he had fallen foul of a cynical and, since it came from within the gay community, to my mind heartless, bit of trickery. It had played out like this.

Hussein had fled to London from Birmingham with a man he thought of as a friend. He told me that one evening he had found this 'friend' waiting for him near Bob's flat. The man had told him that Hussein's father had found out where he was living, and who he was living with. According to the friend, the police had been informed and were even then waiting in Bob's flat for Hussein to come home. If he went in they would both been arrested. So, accompanied by his friend, Hussein had fled down to London. I think Hussein believed the story his friend had told him, but I was a little sceptical: the age of consent for homosexuals was then still 21, but I knew that the police could not arrest either Hussein or Bob unless there was evidence of them sleeping together.

I also told him that since he was over 18, there was nothing in the law to stop him living at Bob's flat. He then told me the rest of the story, which was when I realised he had been very badly taken advantage of by his so-called friend.

As soon as they arrived in London this 'friend' had introduced him to several men, telling him to go off with them. He advised Hussein do as little as possible in terms of sex, but get as much money from them as he could. Some friend, I thought: to turn this handsome young man into a rent boy. Hussein said he hated doing this, but he had to get some money. When I asked him where he was living he said: 'Nowhere: I have slept rough for several nights now'.

I talked to him for a while longer. I didn't entirely believe all that he told me, but there was something about him. Had I met him some time before, while I was still with Steve, I would probably have given him some money, some good advice and wished him luck. But for about the first in my life I had reached a stage where I was going home to an empty house. I told Hussein he could come home with me and – just as I had told Steve – that there were lots of jobs going in Slough. I told him he could sleep in the spare bedroom and look after me and the house until he found a job.

On the way home he asked me to stop, saying he had to pick up some things. He said, he would be only a few minutes. He went off down an alleyway. I waited for 15 minutes and then I thought, 'Oh well, that's that.' I was just about to drive off, when Hussein came running to the car, carrying some clothes and a pair of shoes. I thought, so much for him saying he was sleeping rough. I didn't question him on that, but I was a little suspicious. On the way home I told him that if he was straight with me, he would be okay, but if not he'd be out.

When we got home, I showed him into the spare room and then went to bed. I was just dropping off to sleep, when he got into bed with me. Nothing was said and nothing happened that night, apart from a cuddle – we both, for very different reasons, needed the comfort of another person's body to go to sleep beside. The following day was a Sunday, so we spent the day talking and getting to know more about each other. It was plain to me that he was quite fond of Bob, and was worried about him.

I asked him how old Bob was, and when it emerged that he was middle-aged I realised that Hussein was one of those quite rare younger homosexuals who liked older men. Young men who are attracted to those twice or three times their own age are called gerontophiles. I have known quite a few over the years and I've noticed that almost all of them had a problem where their father was concerned: either they did not grow up with one in the family home or the father had died when they were at an impressionable age. Often they would have had a stepfather who they did not get on with.

I appreciate that this is an unscientific study, but one of the benefits of being as old as I am, and having a lifetime's experience of the gay scene, is the overview it gives of the human dynamics to be found within the relationships forged there. Whether or not the absence of a male paternal role model is a factor in these young men being gay or not, I cannot know. But it is my experience that the 'father figure' complex has applied to five of my seven long-term gay relationships – all of whom were with much younger men. Rodney, my first lover had a stepfather; John's father was more than old enough to be his grandfather; Michael's father was terminally ill and did not treat him very well, and died when Michael was very young. It is anecdotal evidence – of course it is – but something that would, I am sure, be borne out by proper scientific study.

Hussein's history certainly fitted the pattern I have discerned. His family were from Kashmir, the northwestern part of the Indian subcontinent, which is under Pakistani rule. His father had been in England for many years before his family joined him: Hussein was eight years old when he arrived in this country.

Culture is important to Asian communities in Britain. It can be both a force for tremendous good and simultaneously place great strain on children growing up in some families. Hussein's father was a councillor and quite an important man in his community, and with that came responsibilities to traditional Pakistani culture.

Hussein knew that there would eventually be a great deal of pressure on him to get married: he was obviously scared of his father and of his very extended family finding out where he lived, or about his lifestyle. He warned me that I would be in danger if they found out about us, just as he had feared for Bob. He most certainly didn't want to go back to Birmingham.

I told Hussein that he should ring Bob. But he said he was scared to do that and that Bob would be angry with him. Eventually I persuaded him to let me make the call. I had put myself 'in the man's shoes' and I was sure I knew how he felt. The moment I spoke to Bob, and started to talk to him about Hussein, I knew I had done the right thing: the relief in his voice was plain to hear. Young people can be so thoughtless – they just do not realise the deep mental agonies they cause to those who care about them when they just suddenly and unexpectedly disappear.

By arrangement Bob came down the next day to Windsor by coach. All three of us met up at a restaurant. Then the true facts emerged about what had happened. Hussein's so-called friend had managed to gain the trust of both of them and to get a key to Bob's flat. When Bob was at work he had stripped it of all its valuables.

He then told Hussein the story about the police to make it look as if Hussein had been responsible for the theft. And on top of all that, he took him to London and set himself up as the young man's pimp by putting Hussein on the game. Poor Bob was not only very hurt, having helped Hussein a great deal and being very fond of him: he also quite understandably believed Hussein had stolen from him.

And so it came to decision time: what should we all do now? Hussein said that he was uncertain about what to do and my heart sank a little. I realised that I had become very fond of him. Then Bob said the words that made me admire him very much (and indeed since that day he has always been a close friend). He said to Hussein: 'You had better stay with George. It will be a lot better for you with him than with me – and also safer for you to be down here in Slough'.

Bob was a supply landlord to many of the very large pubs in Birmingham (it's the public house equivalent of being a supply teacher). The demands of his jobs meant that he would often have to live-in on pub premises for two weeks at a time. He evidently saw that, given Hussein's difficult family position (and the potential threat that it represented to his safety), living with me in Slough was a much more responsible option – even though it must have hurt him to part from Hussein. But we promised to keep in touch and since I often had to go to Birmingham on business, whenever possible I would call in and see him. Sometimes Hussein would come with me and we would stay the weekend with Bob. At other times Bob would come and stay with us during his holidays.

We had been living together for several months – and had become lovers – when the issue of Asian culture came up again. Hussein said he needed to go to Kashmir to see his relatives, especially his grandfather. I was very uneasy. I had been warned that if he returned to Kashmir there was a real risk his extended family might keep him there and marry him off.

It was, I think, fortunate that I had by now had experience of travelling widely in Pakistan. I knew the ropes a bit and, most importantly, knew who to contact. I told Hussein that as soon as he landed he should go into the capital city, Islamabad, and make an appointment to see the British Consul. I had been there several times on business and knew that it would be vital for the young man to lodge his passport and return ticket with a contact of mine there. I knew, too, that this contact would understand the situation.

But youth is headstrong and Hussein didn't listen to me. He must have told his relatives his flight number and the time he was arriving. They met him at the airport and took him straight to his old home in Kashmir. They also took away his passport and return ticket.

And then he became very ill. Neither of us had thought of the need to have immunisation injections, after all he was going 'home'. But of course he was just like any other British person having lived here for more than 12 years – and had limited immunity (if any at all) to the local diseases.

Hussein's visit to Kashmir happened at a time when we had booked to go together on holiday. With him away I had decided to go alone. I have to say that I didn't enjoy it very much – and my mood of gloom did not lessen when I got back home. I found a pitiful letter from Hussein pleading with me to help him get back to England

I had no idea what to do. Should I go out there and try to rescue him? It didn't seem the safest course – for either of us. Hussein stressed in his letter that I should not write to his family address: instead he gave me the name and address of a contact that he could trust. I wrote back telling him – via his contact – to do all he could to find his passport and return ticket.

It took almost three months before he managed to retrieve them. I received a letter telling me that he was coming home and giving me the date and flight number. I went to the airport to meet him. I waited at the arrivals gate, desperate to catch sight of him. I waited and I waited. There was no sign of Hussein. I phoned the immigration department to see if they were detaining him for any reason, though I couldn't see why they should since he had a British passport. They weren't: nobody seemed to know where Hussein had got to. Eventually I drove home very despondent. As I turned into my road I thought I saw something white suddenly disappear into our gateway.

When I got to the front door I felt a pair of arms around me from behind: it was Hussein, wearing the traditional Asian all-white *shalwar kameez*. Somehow we had missed each other at the airport and he had made his own way home. When we got indoors and I held him in front of me. I could see a light in his eyes: it was the light of love.

I had been in love with Hussein for some time; now I could see without any shadow of doubt that he was with in love with me. If you have experienced that feeling – be it with a man or a woman – you'll know just how wonderful it is.

Hussein got a job at a local fast food restaurant. He did very well and was soon promoted as assistant manager. I also taught him to drive (with great difficulty: never, ever try to teach your lover to drive – it always ends in tears). He saved his money, bought a brand new car on hire purchase and religiously made every payment until the debt was cleared. When I moved home, he moved with me. It seemed we were set for life.

But one day he flashed his smile – the same one which had first attracted me – at a man who was on holiday in Britain. He came from Lebanon and Hussein started meeting and then falling in love with him. The man was about 45 years old and, since he lived thousands of miles away in another largely Muslim country, the affair was doomed from the start. But Hussein was smitten and they wrote to each other regularly.

Lebanon was, at that time, one of the most dangerous places on earth. The bitter and internecine fighting between rival Muslim, Christian and Israeli-backed militia had turned its capital, Beirut, into the hostage centre of the world. Which is why, when Hussein insisted on going over there, all of us who knew him were desperately frightened for his safety. Fortunately, the hostilities had just come to an end, and Hussein returned unscathed. But when his lover came back to England for a second holiday the affair fizzled out. It left Hussein very confused: he told me he did not love me any more, but that he did not want to leave our home.

Hussein stayed with me, sharing a bed with me for almost another year. Perhaps some of you reading this will find the situation strange (though I know many married heterosexual couples who stay and even sleep together long after the light of love has dimmed in each other's eyes). But in my case the arrangement served a very useful purpose: it helped me to get Hussein out of my system and it spared me the hurt of seeing him pack his bags and move out.

We had no sex during that time, but we still cuddled each other in bed and often gave each other a hug during the day. This, I think, is what happens with many relationships, gay or straight: the important thing is the companionship, the helping and looking after each other, sharing the housework, the cooking and shopping and having someone to talk to at the end of the day. Perhaps the difference in homosexual lives is that we are able to be a bit more honest. So Hussein and I (and many other couples in similar situations) were able to talk frankly about any casual sex we each might have.

I didn't blame Hussein for falling out of love with me: how can you blame someone for something like that? It is something that can happen at any time. But my 90-plus years on this planet have taught me one thing above all else: if you love someone you should tell them at least once every day. And that I did.

During the time that Hussein was still living with me, but we were no longer lovers, I had a very short relationship with a chap named John who turned out to be an alcoholic and drug addict. I tried my best to help him, but he was dishonest and was often violent.

Some time after the last time I saw him I was with Hussein in a London pub at Notting Hill Gate. John was there and saw us together. Hussein had met him and quite understandably didn't like him. We left the pub and I walked ahead to the car, when I heard a scuffle behind me, I turned around and saw that John had attacked Hussein from behind. Hussein was on the ground; John had kicked him. I confronted John and after a few blows knocked him to the ground. And then I lost control, kicking John very hard in the ribs while he was on the ground.

I was always taught that you should never kick a man when he is down. My mind cleared and I remembered this. I instantly regretted what I had done (as I have ever since). But I would plead extenuating and mitigating circumstances, for John had attacked the man I realised was still in love with. It was just that Hussein was no longer in love with me. However, our lives were destined to be intertwined for some time to come.

FOURTEEN

As the 1980s came to an end I was 66 years old. The business was still going and I wasn't ready to retire, but it was time to sort out my pension. I duly arranged to convert it to an annuity and was delighted to discover that, with interest rates being sky-high thanks to the economic mess caused by a global economic crisis two years earlier, I was henceforth assured a very comfortable annual income from my investment. It allowed me to travel more, and the trips that I took would result in a series of coincidences that would affect the rest of my life.

On the romantic front, though, life remained somewhat less bright. I had met the man who would become the sixth love of my life, but it was a seemingly complex relationship. During the time that Hussein had not come back from his visit to Kashmir I was very down. A friend took pity on me and said: 'You can't go on like this, he might never come back. Why don't you go to The Quebec?'

I had never heard of the place and was surprised, albeit pleasantly, to discover that it was a pub at Marble Arch frequented by older gays and the younger men who were only attracted to this type. As in the heterosexual lifestyle, the great majority of gay men go for men their own age or younger. The average age of those that crowd the many gay pubs which have (thankfully) blossomed in London is about 30. If a much older man like myself goes to these pubs – which sometimes we do – we feel a little out of place and are usually completely ignored by those in there. For the older homosexual there is the additional disadvantage that the music in these places is always so loud you can't have a comfortable conversation with anyone.

Upstairs at The Quebec turned out to be very different. It is quite large, very nicely decorated and the music is never too loud. On a busy evening there would be at least 150 men aged from 19 to 90, with another 100 downstairs in the small and noisy disco.

There are men from all walks of life and all income brackets, men whom not one, except for a very small handful, would be recognised as gay. All are birds of a feather, wanting only to be at ease, in a friendly relaxed atmosphere: most are not particularly looking for a pick-up.

It was about a year after Hussein and I ceased to be lovers and I was in The Quebec. I was dressed in a dark suit, having been that afternoon to the funeral of a dear friend of mine who had died of Aids. And it was there, and then, that David smiled at me.

David was about 25 with an attractive oriental look. He

told me that his father, who was from Malaysia, was dead and that his English mother was a nurse living in south Wales. He was living with an uncle in Woking. He travelled into London each day for the degree course he was doing.

We were very much attracted to each other and, as things progressed, he spent several weekends at my home as well as going with me on sailing trips aboard *Woody*. When he first arrived at the house I told him I had a lodger, which was the truth: Hussein was no longer my lover – we had stopped sleeping together and he paid for his board and lodging.

But David was suspicious. He annoyed me by not believing me, was unpleasant towards Hussein and wanted me to tell him to leave. This caused some friction between us. I spoke to some of my friends about it and they surprised me by saying that they understood how David felt.

I have never believed in jealousy and possessiveness in the gay life. If there is an arrangement to have an 'open' relationship then so long as there is complete trust and openness between you, where is the problem? I had told David that Hussein and I were no longer lovers and that I always remained friends with my ex-lovers. Shouldn't that be enough?

Nonetheless, Hussein and I had a talk and we decided he would move out. I felt so sorry for I knew how he loved the house and the garden, which he still worked on a lot. I had a large pond, and in it were koi carp that we had chosen and reared together. But, things being what they were, I had to be practical. Hussein duly moved into a tiny room in Slough, only about twice the size of the single bed which filled it.

Life has taught me much, but one of the key lessons I have

learned is that there is a great deal of difference between being 'in love' with your lover and simply loving him. For your lover to be 'in love' with you is to be in the best of all possible worlds; but for one partner to feel more strongly than the other can be the worst of the worst. And I was not 'in love' with David, but he was very much 'in love' with me – and obsessively so.

Naturally, I was flattered. Here was I, two and a half times his age; David was still trying to find his way in life, still a student existing on a £10,000 grant from Barclays Bank. To have him share my life was delightful – up to a point.

He enjoyed sailing but took no interest in the house, the garden or the fish. And after a turbulent 18 months together his love for me had burnt itself out – just at about the time I started to fall in love with him. Such are the ways of the heart. He met an American in The Quebec (of course) and fell for him. When his new love went back to the States, David courted him on my telephone. When he finally left me I found myself staring at a very large phone bill.

I visited Hussein several times in his boxroom; unsurprisingly, he was not very happy there, so when David left he moved back in. We made an arrangement, whereby he would buy all the food and I would pay all the other bills. He loved working in the garden, looking after the fish, cooking on the Aga and, as neither of us were natural loners, it worked very well.

But some time later the pressure on him to get married became overwhelming. It is the custom in his community for the eldest son to marry first. His younger brother had already met his own bride-to-be and wanted to wed, but could not do so until Hussein married. Hussein was, as more gays than straights are, I think, very close to his mother. She, apparently, had to hold her head down in shame as she walked down her street because her eldest son was not yet married. Her husband, Hussein's father, treated her badly and blamed Hussein. Ultimately he gave in.

I was invited to the wedding and, seeing that I would be the only non-Muslim there, a mutual friend of ours called Geoff was invited to keep me company. The wedding took place in two large halls each holding about 200 people and they were both full: all the males, including the groom, were in one hall and all the females, including the bride, in the other.

No one except the groom went into the other hall and even then it was only for a short while. There did not seem to be any ceremony, except whatever took place very briefly during Hussein's visit to the other hall. During the three hours that we were there Hussein sat together with his best man and about a dozen other important people at the top table. Occasionally someone would press some money into Hussein's hand a bit secretively: I watched discretely and saw that this was as much as £40 or £50.

Apparently the whole affair was an excuse for a huge get-together to chat and to give some money to the groom. Hussein told me later that his father collected most of it, a sum which must have amounted to a couple of thousand pounds. Hussein did not see a penny of that. I thought to myself, 'No wonder they wanted him to get married!'

I asked Hussein if anyone had wanted to know who Geoff and I were, and why we had appeared at this very traditional

Muslim wedding. 'Oh yes,' he said, 'I told them you were my landlord and Geoff was your chauffeur.' So much for our relationship, I thought – Hussein and I had lasted for seven years and I was destined to go down as the man who rented him a flat.

The end of my relationships with David and Hussein left me more than a little depressed. 'Travel,' I said to myself, 'travelling will get them out of your system.'

I had been all over the world by then and I scratched my head for a while, wondering where to go. But I remembered that when I'd flown to Australia a few years before, the airline had asked me which route I wanted to take and at which cities I would like to make the required number of stops. There were three options: Hong Kong, Singapore and Bangkok. I had chosen the first two and now, I decided, Thailand was the place to go to get David and Hussein out of my system. I booked a package holiday the next day.

When I arrived in Bangkok I went straight to the most famous and the largest gay sauna in the world. *Babylon* has 1,000 lockers, and at times they are all full. It has a large balcony where you can have food and drink, and it overlooks beautiful gardens that belong to the Austrian Embassy.

In was here that I met Eigg (pronounced 'egg'). He was 30 years old and had the most wonderful ''come to bed' smile. We talked for some time over a cold drink and then he said he would like to come back to my hotel, so I invited him back for dinner.

Although my hotel was only about a mile away, it took us over an hour to get there, through traffic that was at that time about as bad as you will find anywhere in the world.

After dinner we walked out for a drink. I told him that I

would be leaving in the morning on the hotel bus for Pattaya. He could come with me I suggested, and he said he could get some time off work. He would need to go to his home for some clothes, but said that it would not be worth going directly as it would take him three hours.

So at four the next morning he was up, dressed and off to his home on a motorbike taxi, and back again with some belongings in just over half an hour, and back into bed with me. So far, I thought, so good.

At the hotel at Pattaya they only charged me a small amount extra for him to stay with me for the two weeks; there was a large double bed in the room anyway. Eigg was a great help: he knew the town and all the best restaurants. I quickly discovered that there are no taxis in Pattaya, only converted pick-up trucks that have two bench seats in the back, seating 10 or 12 people at a crush. It costs 10 baht to anywhere in the town – around 20 pence. Every day Eigg and I would go to the beach in a 'baht bus', have breakfast in a café and then head to the section that was gay.

There are gay beaches all over the world, and I have visited many of them. Maspalomas in the Canaries is probably the most popular. It is a perfect sandy beach about a mile long with a large section recognised as gay. There are also at least 20 gay bars in the nearby town. These cater for all tastes: leather, disco, porno as well as some ordinary gay bars. A few will be where the older men go and there they will find a fair number of younger men who will only be attracted to those of twice or three times their own age.

But I found that Thailand had a very different – and much less frenzied – feel. I had a wonderful two weeks with Eigg in Pattaya – relaxing all day on the beach with drinks, then taking another baht bus back to the hotel. In the evening, after a rest and maybe a swim in the hotel pool, we would go out for a meal. Perhaps this is what lulled me into a false sense of security.

While on the beach I found myself on my own most of the time: Eigg was off chatting to his Thai friends and so I started talking to another Englishman, relaxing just as I was. It turned out that Eric was born the same year as me; he said he was an English teacher who subsidised his visits to Thailand by teaching English to the Thais.

We chatted happily to each other for several days before I said: 'By the way, where do you live back home?' The surprising answer was Burnham, in Buckinghamshire. It turned out we both lived in the same small village in England. We agreed to get together when were returned home, and I thought very little more of it. I could not have known that this chance encounter would lead to me going to dinner with royalty.

I became very fond of Eigg during our fortnight together. Occasionally I would tell him that I fancied a quiet evening in the hotel and encouraged him to go out and enjoy himself. I would give him some money and was delighted to see that he never came back very late and always put some money back on the side, explaining that he hadn't spent it all.

I made enquiries about getting Eigg over to England. But the more I looked into it the more impossible it seemed it would be. However, I told him I had become very fond of him and that I would be back. On our last night together we returned to Bangkok. He took me to a hotel and enjoyed our last dinner together. When we had finished Eigg said that he wanted me to meet some of his friends in the hotel lounge.

There were about six of us, and we sat having drinks and very pleasant conversation. Then Eigg excused himself to go to the toilet. After about 20 minutes he had not returned and I went to look for him. There was no sign of him, so I went up to the room where we were to have spent our last night together. His small suitcase had gone; on the side was my expensive camera and my suitcase, but nothing was missing except Eigg. I was utterly disconsolate and spent a far from happy last night in Thailand.

The next morning it got worse. I was taken to the airport by the hotel bus and arrived nearly three hours before the flight, instead of the regulation two. I presented my ticket folder – which I had not touched since checking in at Heathrow – to the airline clerk. She took it, looked in it and then asked for my ticket, the return leg of my package flight. It should have been safely tucked in the wallet, but it was not there. I was astonished, and not a little nervous. I was convinced that if it was not where I thought it should have been then it must have been removed in London together with the outgoing half.

The check-in clerk became very official; she refused to accept this suggestion and demanded that I search for the ticket in my luggage. My suitcase had been through the security scanner and had been bound with a metal strap. An official had to be summoned to bring the case back to the check-in, the strap was cut and then I was told to search the case while he stood over me.

By this point I was not in the best of moods, and I became very angry telling them that at no time did I, nor would I, put my ticket in my suitcase. I stormed back to the check-in desk demanding that they fax London for confirmation that

I had paid the return fare and to check at that end. I could not see for the life of me why there should be such a great problem, for all the details of my booking were on the computer screen in front of the clerk.

It took an age before someone got round to sending a fax to London. All this time I was stood on one side while the rest of the passengers were checked in. Then back came the reply. It was not, apparently, possible for my ticket to have been removed at Heathrow. I was informed in a very officious manner I would have to pay again. I presented my gold card and was told 'that will be £950'. I said: 'I don't want a return ticket – I'm never coming back to Thailand'. The check-in clerk shook her head and emphasised: 'That is the single fare.'

I had purchased a package deal that had included a return flight, all hotels for two weeks, plus transport to and from Pattaya and the airport for just over £1,000. But now I was told that £950 was the price of getting home. By this time two hours had gone by. I was feeling exhausted so, with a very bad grace, I paid up resolving to sort the whole sorry mess out when I got back to London. But it wasn't over yet. I was told I must go to the police station at the airport and make out a report as to why I had 'lost' my ticket.

I protested, explaining I had bought another return ticket – so why would I need to do that? At first I refused to go, but I was given no option: the clerk would not give me my boarding card until I did. I was escorted to the police station about a quarter of a mile away, where I was plonked down in front of an officer who did not even look up for some time. When he did finally deign to look at me he said he had no idea why I had been brought to him. I told him what I had been made to do, trying not to show my anger too much. Perhaps it was my previous experiences – almost all unfavourable – with the police in Britain, but I was thoroughly fed up with the humiliating treatment I was being given.

Finally he put a piece of paper in front of me and I wrote down what I knew must have happened to the ticket. He took a long time looking at this: it was now getting near to take-off time and I could see my £950 heading off with the plane. I told the Thai policemen this, but it didn't seem to register. Eventually he gave my escort a piece of paper and I was led back to the check-in desk.

At last! Feeling weak from exhaustion and thirst, I rushed off to the boarding gate. It was another quarter of a mile away and before I was halfway there it was time for my flight to depart. If I missed the plane there was not another for two days – and they were all booked up any way.

Fortunately there was a 15-minute delay. I arrived at the gate soaked in sweat and sagging at the knees. I was brusquely told off for being late and that they were about to unload my baggage. On falling into to my seat I asked a stewardess for a much-needed drink. I was told to belt up – literally and metaphorically – because we were about to take off. I was not, it is safe to say, a happy passenger.

On arrival at Heathrow 12 hours later the aircraft hooked up to the extending passenger bridge. But before the doors were opened there was an announcement over the speaker system. 'Would a Mr George Montague please contact a senior airline official as he leaves the aircraft.'

'Oh God,' I thought, 'will this never end?' I was taken gently by the arm and led to a small lounge. Although I was exhausted, I was aware that this person was apologising all the time, saying how sorry the airline was. We sat down and he explained that – just as I had suggested back in Bangkok – the check-in girl at Heathrow had inadvertently taken out my return ticket together with my outgoing one. It was, he assured me, the first time this had ever happened: he refunded my gold card and handed me a letter of apology together with instructions to claim VIP treatment the next time I travelled with the airline.

I looked him straight in the face and said coldly and clearly: 'I shall never be going to Thailand again. But you *will* hear from my solicitors.'

And in one way, I was right. I sued the airline and, after rejecting their first two offers, accepted my solicitor's advice to settle for £400, plus costs, in compensation.

But in another, far more important, way I was completely and utterly wrong. Because although I had absolutely no intention of going back to Thailand at that point, it would one day become my home from home. And the man with whom I would finally, and wonderfully, fall in love would be a Thai.

FIFTEEN

Back home, still cursing Thailand and the airline, I settled back into the routine of being a single gay pensioner. I celebrated my 70th birthday and the fact that I had now been driving, accident-free, for half a century without ever having passed a British driving test.

I decided that it was time for me to cut down on my workload and so semi-retired from my beloved pattern-making company. I spent the ensuing free time on renovating the large house I had bought and gradually bringing its gardens under control.

But there was something missing: love – obviously, for every man needs that – but also companionship. I decided to look up Eric, the man I had met on the beach in Pattaya and who, in one of those bizarre coincidences, lived very close to me. It proved to be an auspicious decision.

Eric told me that he was a friend of a Colonel in the Nepalese army who was the chaperone of Prince Nirajan, the second son of the King of Nepal. He was 17 years old and at Eton College – itself just down the road. On more than one occasion, Eric told me, he had been invited to the Colonel's home for dinner with the Prince. He had always wanted to return the invitation, but his house was small and not at all suitable to entertain His Royal Highness. Between us we decided my large house would be the ideal place. Eric said he would do all the cooking and cover all expenses.

I have always loved entertaining (and for that matter cooking as well). I said I would be pleased to help him out – and that I would do the cooking. At a loose end in my life, as I then was, I enjoyed preparing a special four-course meal.

The great day arrived and His Royal Highness Prince Nirajan Bir Bikram Shah Dev turned out – despite his blue blood and privileged upbringing – to be a very ordinary and rather likeable lad. The conversation ranged far and wide throughout the meal, and for another couple of hours in the lounge afterwards.

I noticed that Eric constantly addressed the Prince as 'Your Royal Highness', but I found it very difficult to address a 17-year-old old boy like that. It was, perhaps, a lingering trace of the resentment I had felt as a child at the way the rich and powerful gentry had treated my parents. Still, the evening passed off very well, and as the Colonel prepared to take his charge back to Eton the Prince told me that if ever I got to Kathmandu, the capital of Nepal, I was to call at the palace to see him.

As I went to bed that night I wondered if I would ever do so. Certainly, George Montague had come a long way from his humble beginnings – a lad who left school at 14, barely able to read and write – if he could sit down with royalty and then be invited to call in on a Prince. And I very well might have done so, for it would not be long before I travelled east again, had fate not laid a tragic hand on the Nepalese royal family.

In 2001, Nirajan's elder brother and the heir to the throne of Nepal shot to death most of the Royal family – including my one-time dinner guest – before turning the gun on himself. It was, I think, a salutary reminder that wealth and privilege do not always lead to happiness.

But what of my own happiness? Not all was rosy on that front: the economic slump in 1995 and 1996 had hit my company very badly. We had also lost a couple of our most experienced men to retirement. I was by now 74 and still willing to carry on had it been practical – but, frankly, it wasn't. We were tied in to a cruelly demanding lease on the premises and struggling to find the work to sustain it. After much consultation with my accountant I decided to put the company into voluntary liquidation. It was not easy; most businesses that go into liquidation do so because their assets are less than their liabilities. We were not bankrupt, just running out of steam.

With the help of our accountant and liquidator, I managed it. I was friendly with most of my suppliers, and – having had creditors of my own go bust and fail to pay their bills – I was determined to ensure that my suppliers were properly looked after. On the day the company went into liquidation I went round and personally gave them all a cheque, telling them to pay it in straight away.

In the end the business was taken over by my long-time

right-hand man, who had been with me for 30 years. It was just reward for all he had put into the company, but it was, too, a sad day to see the Montague name taken down from above the premises.

All in all, 1997 wasn't looking like the best of years. The one bright spot on the immediate horizon was the election, after 13 years of Conservative rule, of a Labour government. I wasn't an avid follower of politics, more an instinctive Labour voter, but I knew that Tony Blair, before he became Prime Minister, had spoken out in the House of Commons in support of people like me. 'Homosexuality,' he had said, 'is not something you decide to be: it's just something you are.' I couldn't have put it better myself and perhaps, just perhaps, I thought to myself, we might see a little more compassion and a little less of the ant-gay rhetoric which had marked out the years of Tory government.

Not only was the horribly discriminatory offence of gross indecency still on the statute books (and still, shamefully, being applied by police), but we had also, in those years, seen the Clause 28 controversy. The government had forced local councils effectively to class us as second-class citizens in the place where such discrimination could do most harm: schools. Clause 28 of the 1986 Local Government Act instructed local education authorities that they 'shall not intentionally promote homosexuality, or publish material with the intention of promoting homosexuality'. For good measure it also made it an offence to 'promote the teaching...of the acceptability of homosexuality as a pretended family relationship'.

I think those last three words – 'pretended family relationship' – were the most spiteful legal language introduced into Parliament since the Labouchère

Amendment back in Victorian times. And so Tony Blair's apparent commitment to equal treatment for homosexuals was very, very welcome. But even after more than half a century as a gay man I little realised how entrenched homophobia was in Britain – or how the forces of privilege would fight to block much-needed reform of the law.

And then something happened to turn the promise of light into the real thing; and it was blinding. It was 24 June 1997: I will remember the date for the rest of my life – because that was when, after 75 years on this planet, I finally met the love of my life.

I went, that day, to the good old Quebec at Marble Arch. I had been without any sort of lover for many months and was still enjoying the rest which came with that along with finally retiring from the business. When I opened the pub doors I had no intention of picking up anyone, much less of falling in love. I was simply going for a drink with many of my gay friends who I always saw there.

I was facing the door and glancing at those who came in (as one does) while chatting to a friend when suddenly, there in the doorway, walking towards me was one of the most good-looking young men that I have ever seen in my life. He was looking straight at me with such a beautiful smile: I saw instantly that he was from Thailand. He walked towards me still smiling without taking his eyes off me; I was captivated instantly. But then he kept on walking, past me and deeper into the pub. Yet, miracle of miracles, he kept looking back at me.

My friend grinned and said: 'I think you've scored! I'd better leave you or else he will think I'm your boyfriend.' He left me standing on my own. The new and beautiful stranger had bought a drink by this time; he came up to me and we exchanged names. He told me his name was Somchai and that he was only going to be here in England for two more weeks.

I told him I lived in the country 25 miles outside London and straight away he asked: 'Can we go back to your place?' Within five minutes he had finished his drink and we were on the road back to my home. We spent the weekend together during which time I fell in love with Somchai. I'm sure that is the quickest I've done that, but then again, at my age there is no time to waste.

Somchai told me that he was working for Statoil, the Norwegian State owned oil/gas company in Bangkok as a market analyst: he was a graduate with a Masters degree from a Norwegian university. That week he was attending a conference in London and he had to be at Oxford on the Sunday evening to register for a training course, which would last for another week. I said I would take him in my car, which meant we could have another night together. I got him to the hotel where the course was to be held by eight o'clock on the Monday morning: we exchanged phone numbers promising to ring each other sometime during the week. That 'sometime' turned out to be every night.

The following weekend we were again at my home when we suddenly realised that it was Gay Pride week. There was to be a very large gay gathering at Clapham Common that Saturday afternoon. We set off in the car but found we could not park anywhere near one of the entrance gates. We could see thousands on the pavements walking from an underground station towards the Common, so we managed to park the car and joined the walkers. How far we have come, I thought. How long ago does it seem that homosexuals were reviled and lived in a constant state of terror. Now we can not only speak freely about our love, we can take to the streets to demonstrate it. But above all I felt happy and proud to walk with Somchai, arm in arm, in public.

Somchai and I stayed together for the rest of the next week getting to know each other before he had to go back to Thailand. During the next six weeks we phoned each other at least four times a week (and in those days it cost a £1 a minute) and wrote loving, tender letters to each other: neither of us will ever part from those letters – just as we will never part from each other.

We had arranged that I would fly out to Thailand to meet him. I smiled as I cast my mind back to my vehement insistence to the check-in clerk at Bangkok Airport that I was never coming back. How little we realise the way that fate changes our lives for us. And so I flew out to meet my lover and stayed in Thailand with him for three weeks. During that time he resigned from his job, gave up his flat and obtained a post-graduate student's visa so that we could both come back to England together.

But what sort of country was Britain now? It was a question that occurred to me as Somchai and I began our life together in our new home. Thailand is one of the most tolerant places on the planet for gay men and women. He had given up his old life – for me. What sort of welcome would my country extend to him?

On one level things were looking better than they had for a while. True to the promise I had seen in Tony Blair and his government, it introduced a proposal to Parliament that the age of consent for homosexual acts should be brought into line with the law on heterosexual behaviour: a few years earlier the age of consent for gays had been lowered from 21 to 18, but this was still two years later than that for straight people. The new law would bring in a universal age at which people could have sex – 16. The House of Commons passed the law with a huge majority. But then the House of Lords swung into action. This palace – and I use the word correctly – of peers voted down the proposal and thus stopped it becoming law.

The next year, and the year after, the government tried again. Each time the House of Commons – which is to say the MPs who are actually elected by a democratic vote – backed the legislation; each time the unelected peers struck it down. Those campaigning against it did so by raising the despicable spectre of paedophilia: they said they were simply acting to protect children. The leader of the 'no' campaign, Baroness Young, said: 'Homosexual practices carry great health risks to young people.' Well of course they did – but then, so did (and do) heterosexual acts.

The fight between the Houses of Commons and Lords was, in the arcane way of British democracy, a constitutional crisis – who was to rule the country, the elected or the unelected? Finally the government used a constitutional lever to force the law on to the statute book; it eventually received Royal Assent in 2000.

Somchai and I knew very quickly that we were perfect for each other. But his family were in Thailand, while mine were in England. Somchai's father had been killed in a road accident when he was four or five years old; his mother and brothers still lived in the same area where he grew up.

The answer, when it came to us, was simple: have a house in both countries and divide our time between them. Somchai has, in addition to his studies, always been a good businessman with a gift for buying and selling property and we were both well enough off to make the plan work.

And so it did. We found our Thailand home just outside Pattaya, only a short walk from the gay beach. It was then a 10-year-old bungalow in need of a little care and attention. We hired Somchai's brother to renovate and paint everything; he lived about 150 miles away, but on the day work was to start he arrived with seven other workmen and set about the task. They quite literally slept on the job: they worked from first light in the morning until late in the evening, then each night they simply slept on the floor.

It took two weeks – a fortnight in which every inch was refurbished, carpets were ripped up from the bedrooms and beautiful parquet flooring laid down. More men came to put up the guttering, others came to modernise the electrics and still more to service and repair the air conditioning. The front patio was made waterproof and extended to form a carport. The cost was about a quarter of what I would have expected – and they did a truly excellent job.

What made everything even easier for us was that Thailand was happy to welcome me – a *farang*, as foreigners are called – to the country. At the time when Somchai and I decided to spend our lives together Thailand was far more accepting of same-sex couples like us than Britain.

It was possible for heterosexuals to gain entry or to stay together in the UK if they could prove that they had been living together for one year. But for homosexuals there was no such concession no matter how long they had been together. Fortunately – and living up to the promise I had seen in Tony Blair – the government set about changing this. Before too long it brought in rules that made it possible for someone like Somchai to stay in Britain – as long as there was proof of cohabitation in a couple's relationship for two years. And provided he enrolled on a post-graduate course at a recognised university.

Somchai started a folder, keeping all letters, birthday and Christmas cards with the envelopes and the date stamp. He took photographs that proved we were together: pictures of us standing in front of a poster with the date on it. When the millennium dome was half-built, he took a photo with the dome in the background then, when it was finished we did the same thing again. The progress of the dome would help to prove that we had been together for the required period.

We changed all suppliers' accounts into our joint names and all our bank statements and receipts went into the folder. We went to the theatre and concerts at the Albert Hall at least once a month; we kept all ticket stubs and programmes, as well as all boarding cards and plane tickets when we flew anywhere.

Then when the two-year period was almost up we wrote to about 20 friends who had known the pair of us for some time asking them to write a letter confirming that we had been living together as a loving couple for two years. The file was by this time about three inches thick.

Finally we put in our application and waited. And waited. Then, in the autumn when it was getting near the time for us to go to Thailand for six months, we were summoned to an interview at the Home Office in Croydon. The official saw us just before lunch, but she told us that there was no chance of our application being considered before the spring of the following year. We asked her about the possibilities of applying while we were in Thailand. She said there might be a chance of getting the approval via the British Embassy in Bangkok, but this would mean withdrawing our application: worse still, if we went down this route Somchai would have to leave the UK within three weeks.

In the end we realised that we really had no choice, and so we withdrew our British application and as soon as we arrived in Bangkok we resubmitted it at the Embassy. It must have been the first one they had come across, for they were not too sure what to do with it. However after a bit of pressure we received an interview date: 7 January 2000.

On the due date we were at the British Embassy at eight in the morning and were quite quickly shown into a little interview room. I was told that they only interviewed the applicant, and politely, but firmly, told to wait in an anteroom. Somchai, in fear and trepidation, stayed on alone to answer the questions. The only time that he faltered was when the woman conducting the interview asked why he was in a partnership with a man so much older than himself. Like the great majority of people she had presumably not heard of the term gerontophile.

Still, she seemed quite knowledgeable about us, and told Somchai that she had taken our file home the evening before and spent most of the evening reading it. And then, after no more than 20 minutes, she told him we had been successful. It meant that Somchai could come and go in and out of the UK as often as he pleased, and could work legally.

It was a tremendous relief: we were now able to give each other the support and love that sustains any couple. And before long I was to need Somchai's support as never before.

In 2002, at the age of 68, my wife died of a severe stoke. Vera and I were married for over 20 years; and although we had been living apart almost as long, her death came as a great shock.

There had been some bitterness on her part when I first left her and I agonised for a long time afterwards. I felt terribly guilty but, over time, I had gradually been able to see very clearly that what I did was right for her. Vera loved me so much that she would never have told me to leave – she knew and accepted the fact that I was gay, that our sex life together was over and that I had male lovers but that, on its own, wasn't enough to kick me out.

Our relationship had changed into one of companionship but we both knew that I could no longer give her the attention and the fun in life that she deserved. I knew that she needed to meet someone who could give her the things that I could no longer provide. And, as it turned out, just a few years after we parted she met Harold. Harold was a widower with his own house and car; together they went dancing and on holiday. He became to her what I could not have been and they were together as a couple for 15 years.

She never moved in with him, but they enjoyed their life together and in the years that followed the bitterness Vera had felt on our parting ebbed away. I visited her often, and after Somchai and I became a couple he came with me; she greeted him warmly and as someone who cared for me.

We had planned another visit and were getting ready to go down to see her when my son telephoned to say that Vera had suffered a stroke. Somchai and I rushed down, but instead of seeing her at her home, we saw her on her deathbed. She died three days later without regaining consciousness.

In all their years as a couple I had never met Harold until that day at Vera's hospital bedside. When we arrived he was the only person with her, sitting beside the bed and holding her hand. I said: 'You must be Harold.' And he replied: 'Yes – and you must be George.'

Talking to him I quickly realised that he did not know how serious Vera's condition was. Hospitals – supposed to be places of kindness, attention and healing – have rules that are so downright thoughtless and cruel when it comes to deciding to whom they give out information. Harold, who had been her constant companion for 15 years, was not a blood relative and so not entitled to be given any information whatsoever.

If Harold – who I gathered from our short talk was the retiring type, not one to push himself forward – had told them that he was her common-law husband they would have told him what they later repeated to me and what they had told my son – that Vera had suffered a severe stroke and that if she regained consciousness at all she would be severely disabled. Vera's brother was severely disabled and confined to a wheelchair; she had often told me that she would not want to live like that.

Harold had told me that he had known several people who had suffered strokes who had been unconscious for many days but had subsequently been left with only slight disabilities. He was plainly hoping that would be the case with Vera. But he said that even if her disabilities were severe, she would come to live with him and that he would look after her. Both my son and I were too distraught and upset to explain to Harold the seriousness of Vera's condition.

While writing this I find I am becoming angry, because the same attitude and rules that denied Harold the information he deserved to have also affects gay couples. Homosexuals who have spent decades living together, loving each other and caring for each other, through good times and bad, find that if they end up in hospital in a critical condition they will often be denied the right to visit. The fact that those blood relatives who may not have seen or contacted the patient for many years is allowed is, apparently, irrelevant.

I have seen situations where blood relatives have disowned their son or daughter because of their gayness, then grabbed everything when the person dies, even turning a partner out of the home they shared if the deceased's name was the only one on the deeds or there was no will. And this happens despite the fact that the surviving partner may have shared all expenses including mortgage repayments.

I don't particularly blame those relatives – many people these days will grab whatever they can whenever they can. But in the days after Vera's death I came to question how this could be. How, at the start of the 21st century, could such unfairness and prejudice exist? The law needed to catch up – and that meant civil partnerships that would protect homosexuals, as well as giving them comfort. The government had promised them – but they were still a few years away.

I was proud to be at Vera's funeral with Somchai beside me, and to introduce him to everyone as my partner. But while I have always led the singing at the many funerals I have been to, I was unable to sing a single note at my wife's funeral.

The emotion of the day was one reason. But there was another one too: for two years I had been taking significant quantities of medication every day. Without that medication I would, quite possibly, not even have been at the funeral. You see, two years before we buried Vera I had contracted HIV.

SIXTEEN

I've always liked saunas for the three Ss: the sauna itself, the social side and the sex. You can't do anything in a sauna or steam room except sweat, talk or play about.

I went to my first sauna, in Durban, South Africa, at the end of World War Two, while I was waiting for the boat to take me home. Since then I doubt I have been as long as a month without going to one. You have never been so clean, no matter how many baths or showers you have, than when you leave a good sauna. The sweat just rolls off you, all your pores open up and all the dirt flows out.

After about 15 minutes the heart starts beating faster: I have always believed that this is a good thing (unless of course you have a heart problem) and it has been shown that when used properly, saunas can lower the blood pressure, reduce hormones, assist diabetes and lung conditions and even help to fight off the common cold.

And it's also true that saunas can improve your sex life. And not just for the obvious reasons. Around the world there are certain saunas that operate as places where men (and sometimes women) can meet and enjoy sex. But even in these sexually oriented spots there is a great deal of honest conversation – and it can, under the circumstances, be very stimulating.

I have talked with and listened to the conversations of many hundreds of men who, though they might not admit it, have homosexual desires. Many times I have asked them questions that provoke revealing responses: 'At what age did you discover or admit to yourself that you were gay? What did you do? Were you seduced? Who with?'

The answers I got from many of the middle-aged or older men were frequently remarkably similar: 'I don't know if I'm gay or not. I still live with my wife, I still love my wife, I still have sex with her but not very often; she doesn't seem to want it anymore. I came here to see what a sauna was like. She doesn't know that I come here, and I found that a masturbation here was better than doing it on my own at home. I don't fuck or be fucked, but I've thought about it. Am I gay?'

I think we have got to adjust the definitions of whom we call gay and whom we call straight. The number of men who never have and never will have sex with a woman is relatively small – I would guess no more than two or thee per cent. Then there are men who have tried to go straight but gave in to their urges or discovered that they prefer men. This group is I'm sure very much larger than the first group.

Then come the third group, much larger than the first two, who frequently go to gay saunas and gay cruising areas, usually middle-aged or older men who on the face of it live a normal heterosexual life but who are feeling horny, are not 'getting any' and have found it easier to get a quick 'hand job', 'blow job' or full sex in these locations.

And so, we – that is, Somchai and I – were in the gay sauna in Bangkok. Somchai was, as he usually did, keeping an eye open. 'There's a guy eyeing you up,' he said. He was about Somchai's age, very good-looking and with a preference for older men, just like Somchai.

Before we get to what followed, I think we need to take a moment to discuss the notion of jealousy. I believe fervently that we should stop using the words unfaithful, jealous and possessive. I have been lucky enough to have long-term loving relationships with seven men (including Somchai). I'm sure you will find it hard to believe me when I say I have never experienced jealousy, but it's true. Of course I've been disappointed and sad when the relationships have ended and maybe asked myself, what if anything did I do wrong. But jealousy? No, never. It's illogical to hate the person your lover has gone off with, even if it feels like he has been poached from you.

In the years that Somchai and I have enjoyed together – loving years, good years – there has never been the slightest hint of mistrust, secrecy, possessiveness or jealousy between us. In the gay life open relationships are common. In the straight world it goes on just as much, but it's not often as open. He gets a lot more offers than I do but he rarely takes them up. If I get an offer, it's often Somchai who tells me that I have an admirer and he encourages me. Our love for each other is just as great as – no, considering the pressures, temptations and the sigma and disapproval that still exists to this day, it is even greater than – any other couple I have known.

We have a very open relationship and we think nothing more of 'jumping into the sack with another fuck buddy' than we would of dancing or playing a game of something together. And, if I have ever learned anything from life, I know that you can't have true love without trust. Jealousy is just plain illogical.

Which brings us back to the sauna in Bangkok.

In some of us the sex drive is extremely powerful and remains so well into old age. I was 77 at the time. However, like men many years younger than me, I found that putting on a condom tended to ensure the loss of my erection. These were the days before the widespread availability of the helpful little pills that cure that particular difficulty. And so, when Somchai pointed out the attractive man eyeing me up – and with his blessing – I was tempted. And when it was offered to me, I took the forbidden fruit without a condom.

Tell me: which of the two elements of this story worries you more? Is it the fact that I foolishly had unprotected sex – or the fact that I did so while in a full-time and loving relationship? And, indeed, in front of him?

Sex with someone you love is the most wonderful thing in the world. But, to use an analogy, after a few years, eating egg and bacon for breakfast every day can become a bit boring. Quick sex with a stranger for the first time is exciting. It has nothing to do with loving the person. And if you have an open relationship with complete and immediate openness and honesty, I can tell you that it strengthens a relationship and invigorates the sex life.

No, it wasn't having brief and fairly anonymous sex with

a stranger which was the problem: it was doing so without a condom. As soon as possible both Somchai and I went for an extra check-up at the local hospital. And we were given good news: no infection, an all-clear on the medical front. What we didn't then know is that it takes several weeks for the infection to show. About a month later I became very ill. I was in Pattaya hospital for a few days, then in the best hospital in Bangkok. But having told them I'd been checked out recently and given a clean bill of health they did not check for HIV. And neither did Paddington Hospital in London when I went there after we got home.

My HIV was eventually discovered not by the STD clinic but by the doctor in a very special unit. Because, unlike most people presenting with early HIV symptoms, we knew exactly when I had been infected – and yet had subsequently had a negative test – I was of special interest to him. The information about when I picked up the disease enabled him to put me on a new and experimental regimen of treatment.

Dr Michael Brady was at that time getting ready to conduct a study to see if patients should receive treatment before the condition got worse or only when it became acute. In 2000, the accepted wisdom was to start medical treatment only after a patient's condition reached a certain critical point. I was one of the first to volunteer to be part of an experiment that prescribed a full and aggressive treatment long before it was clinically needed.

I owe Dr Brady my life. Ten years on after this study doctors now know that it is best to hit HIV with the kitchen sink as soon as it is contracted. My treatment proved to be the saving of me and I slowly improved. I was careless, reckless even, in contracting HIV. I knew the risks of unprotected sex – risks that had already claimed so many lives all over the world. I am alive only because of the drugs that came in just a few years before. I have been punished, quite justly so. It left me with neuropathy in my legs and feet, unable to walk for many months and having to be pushed around in a wheelchair by Somchai. I am also dependent on retroviral drugs for the rest of my days.

And I know not just that I was incredibly lucky but that today there are many – far too many – people playing Russian roulette in the way that I did. And many – again, far too many – of them are young. In some parts of the gay community HIV has almost been forgotten, a by-product, perhaps, of the very drugs which saved my life. Too many young gay men now behave as if the treatment is a cure – which it unquestionably is not.

There are now gay pick-up sites on the Internet for people seeking 'bare-back' (as our little world calls unprotected) sex. They are treating HIV as an inconvenience that can be overcome with a quick dose of drugs.

We need to get some perspective. There is no excuse now whatsoever for condoms not being used. Yes, they may dampen the ardour a little (so to speak) but the little blue pills are very cheap. A quick doctor's examination, to ensure the heart is okay, and a prescription, which can be either on the NHS or private, are all you require.

So it's a pill (if you need one) and a condom every time. The luck that I have had all my life, except for this one foolish episode, is still with me. At 91 I am still enjoying life to the full. Even my sex life is okay.

And – lest anyone think that this is nothing more than a

private and personal issue, a decision to be taken by individuals in response to their own particular circumstances – I believe strongly that we, the gay community, need to realise that what we each do about sex has the potential to derail every little bit of understanding and equality which has, finally, been granted to us.

AFTERWORD

As these memoirs are being written I am sitting happily in the warmth of Thailand. The house I share with Somchai is situated just a few hundred yards from a beautiful sandy beach several miles long: the seawater, at body temperature, is always welcoming.

Our village consists of about 40 houses and two very large high-rise condominiums. These funnel the light and a constant sea breeze straight onto our patio. There is a large swimming pool, tennis courts and never fewer than six security guards on duty – all for a service charge of about £100 a year. We also have a maid who comes in five days a week to do all the housework, the washing and the ironing. She even cuts the grass and looks after the garden.

We have turned the smallest of our four bedrooms into a study. Somchai now spends a lot of his time there, working as the (self-employed) breadwinner of our partnership and doing similar work to that he was engaged in when we met and he came to live with me in England. We let our London flat to a company based in Bangkok, one of whose young employees is a long time friend of Somchai's.

And what do I do? I tap away on this computer setting down these memoirs.

Several times over the years I thought about recording the story of my life. When I began there was never any thought in my mind about publishing my memoirs: it was an exerciser – something to keep my mind active. But as the pages mounted up it seemed that there might be a value to others in them. In itself this posed some difficult and fundamental questions. How honest should I be about my life, my sexuality, my relationships and my sex life in memoirs that would then be sent out into the world?

I have never worried about what complete strangers think: in this, perhaps, I am lucky since so many people go through life fearful of the reaction of people who they don't know and are never likely meet. Nor was I concerned about the response of my friends: the reaction of the great majority of friends and acquaintances who might read this would not, I was sure, be one of shock or disgust.

So why did I hesitate? It was, I realised, the potential effect on my family. Writing one's memoirs is a bit like being in the dock: it's 'the truth, the whole truth and nothing but the truth'. In writing it – no, in *publishing* it – would I be causing pain?

In the end I was reassured that my fears were groundless. I've never done anything with anyone I shouldn't have, or without their consent. And as to the sex: well, I hope everyone will try to understand that sex is a small – but vitally important – part of life.

And so the typing began. It was not, of course, a simple process, nor one that always came easily. There were sleepless nights and many doubts. But throughout them I was supported by Somchai.

Fortunately for me, he is my last love and the love of my life. I am as certain as I can be that he will be with me until the day I die, and I am positive that when it comes my date with death will be much later than it would have been without him. And so, after five years together I found I was able to set down the story of a gay man's progress through life.

In doing so, it dawned on me the reason why this might, just might, be important to others. A memoir should tell it as it is and I have tried to set down as true an account of my life as my faculties allow – and of what it has meant to be homosexual over the course of almost 100 years.

I would dearly love to have been able to read just such an account in the days when I went though agony over my sexuality. And I would hope that any religious bigot or homophobe who might read it will have a change of heart and concede that unlike many of them, we who do no harm to anyone deserve and have a right to a little love, happiness and understanding.

And there's the word that drove me forward: understanding. Because throughout my life, and still today, homosexuality has been condemned by religious leaders who should know better, misunderstood and wrongly conflated with paedophilia. These memoirs – the setting down of the who, what, where, why and when of a gay man's progress through almost a century – could have, I realised, a real purpose: to challenge religious homophobia, to draw a clear and unequivocal line between homosexuality and paedophilia, and to campaign for one of the last changes our newly enlightened society needs to make.

After all, who better than I to take on this task? I devoted long years of my life to the church. I was wrongly suspected of being a danger to children. And, as my body weakens, I can see the world from the perspective of other gay men (and women) who are entering their twilight years.

And so, after all you have read of what befell me and how I spent my years on this planet, this final chapter is a plea for tolerance and for true understanding.

So let's start with paedophilia. And let's start with a clarion call that needs to be heard across this land, and far beyond. There is no more connection between homosexuality and paedophilia than there is between heterosexuality and paedophilia.

By chance – or not, who really knows? – this country where Somchai and I avoid the English winter is a good place to start. I have found – and I have said to you – that Thailand is the most tolerant country in the world for homosexuals. But in recent years Thailand has become known as a haven for paedophiles.

Reports in the international press have highlighted the phenomenon of child sex tourism – wealthy westerners (and they are usually westerners) flying in and using their hard currency to obtain young children for sex. In many cases the victims are boys. And these reports are true.

But they also tend to become mixed in with the equally real phenomenon of adult sex tourism – and thereby to blur the perceived boundaries between homosexuals and paedophiles. So let me, in the candid spirit of these memoirs, be honest and tell you about this country I have come to love and the area in which Somchai and I live.

According to the *Bangkok Post* there are 5,000 bars, nightclubs, massage and sauna venues throughout Thailand. These are all male or female brothels, although they may not be officially called that. Spread throughout the large towns and cities – again according to the *Bangkok Post* – there could be as many as a million men and women working as prostitutes: some are full-time sex workers, others work only when they need the money.

In Pattaya, where Somchai and I chose to live, there must be 5,000 women and an equal number of young men all working part-time or full-time in the sex industry. And on a typical walk through the town you will see a great many middle-aged (mostly) Caucasian men, twice or three times as old as the man or woman with whom they are strolling arm in arm, or hand in hand.

One whole street is called Boyz Town. It boasts exclusively gay bars, a gay sauna, and gay restaurants. Did you note the name: 'Boyz'? At first glance (and some reporters rarely seem to bother with a second one) this could indicate under-age sex. But the truth is that it doesn't: it is simply the way young Thai men working in the sex industry refer to themselves and, in turn, are referred to by their customers. They are all adults – all Thais have to, by law, carry an identity card that shows their date of birth. Goaded by the international reports of paedophile tourism, the police regularly check these bars and brothels.

The biggest of these is called – of course – *Boys, Boys,*

Boys: it claims to offer 100 young men to the clientele. Inside in the centre is a large circular stage on which they dance: each wears a very brief pair of underpants and a number on a pin disc. The customers are mostly men – although sometimes there is a woman wanting a toyboy; they sit at small tables and chairs where they pay through the nose for drinks. When a customer takes a fancy to a particular young man he will signal for him to sit next to him. Then, if all is well and they decide to leave, he will call a waiter who comes and makes up his bill. He adds 250 baht (£4) for the young man's time.

Upstairs there are rooms where the man can have sex with his new acquaintance. If he chooses to do so, he will pay extra to the club's management and 500 baht (£8) to the young man for what is called 'short time'. If the customer takes the young man back to his hotel it is 500 baht for short time and a minimum of 1,000 baht (£16) for an all-night stay.

Does this shock you? Reading this are you thinking that this trade is outrageous and should be stopped? If so, I sympathise: I must admit that when I first came here I was saddened by what I found. But read on, please read on.

Unlike the thousands of men who come here from all over the world, almost always on their own, I don't come for the Thai young men. I come because Thailand is my partner's home country and where his family is. His sisters, brother and mother, of whom I am very fond, now consider me as part of the family.

But I am incurably nosy and I have always gone out of my way to speak with these young men for hire, and always asked lots of questions about their lives. And in doing so, I have come to see the sex industry here in a different light.

Poverty here has become a great deal worst since my first visit in 1996. The following year saw the Asian economic slump, with the Thai currency losing one-third of its value: even today this is a poor, poor country. And the two Ps – poverty and prostitution – invariably go together.

It may sound odd, but here in Thailand – and in the gaudy sex-for-hire world of the Pattaya bars and brothels – I am constantly reminded of a saying of Mahatma Ghandi: 'There is enough in the world for everyone's need, but not enough for everyone's greed.' Thailand is very much a land of the 'haves' and the 'have-nots'; there are very many very rich people – and far too much corruption. And so, there is a dilemma. If sex tourism puts food on people's tables and clothes on their backs, is it always wrong?

Here's what I learned from the young men involved in these transactions (they call themselves 'money boys' and therefore so shall I). Once you have read this then, perhaps, it will be time to make up your mind.

The initial introduction into the world of sex for hire for many male money boys is from their friends. Young men go back to their village with a lot of money in their pockets, much of which they give to their very poor parents telling them they have worked hard in restaurants and hotels. They talk to some of their friends who work long hours for a week in the field or a factory to get the same as a money boy gets for going to bed with a gay foreigner for one night.

There is, it appears, a code of conduct among the young men. They are very careful about who they tell what they are doing or what goes on. No one under the age of 18 is told. They are also very careful that their parents do not find out.

Young men in these villages have three choices. The first is to stay with their families where, although they won't starve, they will all be extremely poor. The second is to get a job in the towns and cities where most will be exploited by subcontractors for international companies and will earn barely enough to survive. To their credit, many young Thai men choose this option, but they are unable to make enough money to help their families. The third choice is to take up part-time or full-time sex work as a money boy.

From my experience those that take up this option know exactly what they are getting into. They do nothing they don't want to do. They give as little as they can get away with. And they get as much out of the *farangs* as they can.

They often persuade their customers to fall in love with them, and since many of those they go with are already very old, when they die the boy ends up a baht millionaire. And since the *farangs* come back year after year for more, it doesn't seem that they object to this commercial exploitation.

So: you have read now how the system works. Are you still shocked? Do you still believe that the Thai government should close all these venues and put a stop to foreign men coming here just for sex? If so, I am afraid I disagree with you.

If that were to happen, what would the poor young men do? The eternally smiling faces of Thailand would smile a lot less because they and their families would go hungry. And nothing will change until there is a very great improvement in the global economic situation. Some people look at sex tourism as a form of International Aid, but the simplest reality is that it is the result of inequality in wealth. Before you condemn what goes on you should come to Thailand and see for yourself the poverty that exists here. Is paying for sex so wrong when it alleviates this?

Perhaps my conclusion is based on my history: as you now know I have on several occasions engaged in sex with rents boys (and women prostitutes, too). But after 91 years on the planet I have to ask: what is so wrong with one adult who has the money paying another adult for sex – as long there is no coercion?

What is unquestionably wrong is to allow a perfectly understandable moral objection to Caucasian men renting sexual services from younger Thai men to be conflated with paedophilia. That, sadly, has happened – and I know only too well the devastating consequences of being wrongly tarred with that particular brush.

In case you doubt me, it was while these memoirs were being written that a public figure, an elected councillor no less, stood up and announced: 'All queers are paedophiles.'

Paedophilia is something gay people knew about long before the immense problem (as we have discovered it is) became almost daily news. We hated them: if we found someone amongst our ranks that we suspected had sexual desires for children we would ostracise them.

And yet even today too many people assume all gay men are a danger to children. It makes me despair.

Which brings us to the cause of much of the prejudice and misunderstanding about homosexuality – prejudice and misunderstanding, which, lest you forget, caused the imprisonment and death of men who dared to love other men. It has a name, this cause: and its name is religion.

I was a devout believer in Christianity up until about the age of 60. By then I had devoted a large part of my life to religion and to celebrating God by singing sacred music. I believed and felt the words I was using, just as I did when I read the lessons from the Bible to the congregation at church. I did, it is true, find many of the stories in the Bible hard to swallow. But I was brainwashed and indoctrinated from a young age.

But at the age of 60, by which time I had lost both my parents, and a brother, all of whom I wanted to believe I should see again in an afterlife, I realised that according to the main religions of the world I am a sinner. Most faiths condemn homosexuality: some of the harsher sects even execute gays. Too many churches in too many religions say that sex between man and man is an abomination. And so I stopped being brainwashed and started to think seriously about it all. And I decided that if the church cannot accept me as I am, then no longer could I accept the church.

Tell me (if you can) how, in the 21st century, can we condemn people based on something in the Bible, the Quran or the Torah? On scriptures written so many years ago, by people who – just like many today – did not understand homosexuality, nor ever want to? How can religion condemn those that want to love another person of the same sex? Most humans are not loners like some animals. If God (of whatever faith or persuasion) made us, then why did he arrange it that about 10 per cent of males and seven per cent of females are attracted to someone of the same sex?

Religious leaders tell us that we homosexuals should resist temptation. But what have we done so wrong that such apparently terrible temptation is put in our path? I no longer believe in the religion to which I gave so much of my life. I must have been mad.

Has this final chapter in the memoirs of a long life, fully lived, become a little too acerbic for you? Fine: I shall put aside my soapbox and move on to something a little less challenging – and yet which could enrich the lives of gay men and women as they reach their last years.

Today gay people can legally go on holiday together, visit gay clubs and pubs, stay in gay guest houses and gay hotels: but when it comes to having to go into a care home, we pretty much have to stop being gay. Why? Because care homes for the elderly are some of the last bastions of homophobia.

The vast majority of care homes are full of old straight people, who do not even begin to accept or understand homosexuality. As my age increased and my health diminished I spent some time researching the issue: I discovered that of all the thousands of care homes in Britain none are avowedly gay friendly – and some are openly homophobic. The case of an elderly gay woman makes the point.

This lady had a hip operation and when she received care in her home, she had a carer who gave her a sponge bath at arm's length. The carer wouldn't go near this poor women when she was naked because she knew she was a lesbian.

The demand for the needs of older gay people to be acknowledged is growing as the general ageing population grows. Can it be right to live in a care home where you have to hide your sexuality? To push *Gay News* behind a cushion when anyone comes into your room, or hide a photograph of your partner because you worry about the response from your carer? I had 40 years of living a lie. Now I want to redress that balance and shout from the rooftops that care homes must become gay friendly. It's not that I want exclusively homosexual homes, but I am adamant that a gay person should never have to spend their last years in fear of prejudice and discrimination. I have told Somchai that if the time ever comes when he has to put me into a home it's got to be one that has a lot of other old gay men or I'm not going. Full stop.

And so, at last, I have come to the end of these memoirs. From the age of 25 I have been loved very much and been in love with seven men, two of whom still loved me on the day they died. For many years, the late-40s, 50s and 60s, I hated being gay, I would have given anything, done anything, for a cure. Now that I am in the twilight years of my life and have long since realised there is no such thing as a cure, I am glad to be gay. And I am certain that if I had known then what I know now I would never have got married.

Vera was the one woman I ever loved – and I loved her very much – but however hard I tried it was impossible for me to be 'in love' with her. Vera, my love, mother of my children, I am so sorry.

But there is no question of my ever regretting the years we spent together. I was incredibly lucky to have found a woman who loved me so much, even though it was a love that was impossible for me to return in the true sense of the word. Oh, yes, Vera loved me, despite knowing that I was gay, and she gave me three wonderful children; she stayed with me even after she discovered that I had broken my promise to give up having sex with men; and she enabled me to live the lie that one just had to live in those days.

I am comforted that the last years of her life were a great deal happier than they would have been if I had stayed with her. And, a few years ago, I was comforted too by a letter from Vera's sister.

When she discovered the dark secret of my homosexuality, Doffie had been very critical of me for marrying her beloved sister. And yet, after she came to a party that Somchai and I had thrown, she found it in her to open up her mind and her heart.

Dear George and Somchai

What a splendid party yesterday! Thank you for asking me. I really enjoyed it so much and to find you still full of the old enthusiasm for life. I can't tell you how good it was to meet and talk with your friends and relations. It was an education to find that your gay community are no different to anyone else; I found them pleasant and warm and it's really good that there is no longer any discrimination which should, on reflection, have disappeared many eons ago.

Until next time, take care, keep living, laughing and loving.

Love from Doffie

I owe Doffie my thanks: her letter, particularly given the hostility she once felt towards me and my ilk, has given me renewed hope. And at my age that is no bad thing.

The reason I wrote these memoirs was not to list all the many things I have done in my life, but to make an attempt at getting people to accept – through the story of my life to try and understand homosexuality, and to accept it.

How do you go about getting a heterosexual to understand homosexuality? How do you explain what it is like to be homosexual? By telling the truth – the difficult, uncomfortable bits of truth, as well as those that slip past more easily.

THE OLDEST GAY IN THE VILLAGE

This memoir is who I am. I have committed to the computer's memory everything that I can recall about my life, and in so doing I hope I have shed light on how it came to be that gay men and gay women can speak at last of their loves. I hope, too, that I have pointed at ways that we can still improve our treatment of people like me.

Once upon a long time ago I was the only gay in the village, and – though my neighbours never knew it – I was forced to live a lie. Now I am now the Oldest Gay in the Village, sure and safe in the arms of the love of my life. And I know this, if I know anything at all: love – wherever, however it is found – is the most important thing in life. But love can only flourish openly where there is understanding.

And so, for all my faults and failures, for the frankness and honesty with which these poor pages are set down, I hope that you may come to some understanding. If so, then my work, truly, is done.

ACKNOWLEDGEMENTS

I would like to thank the *Slough Observer*, the *Windsor Express*, and the *Maidenhead Advertiser* for their kind permission to reproduce certain photos in this book. Thanks too go to Clare Christian who first contacted me about my story and who has helped guide me through the publishing process. Finally very grateful thanks go to Tim Tate, the excellent editor who took my words and helped craft them into this book.